From the Vedas to Vinyasa

An Introduction to the History and Philosophy of Yoga

Amy Vaughn, M.A.

Opening Lotus Publications
Tucson, Arizona
ISBN-13: 978-0-69-268339-2

DEDICATION

To my teachers

CONTENTS

ACKNOWLEDGMENTS

For a book like this, it is only appropriate to acknowledge my teachers. The research for this book started over twenty years ago when I took my first class in Eastern Philosophies from a man named, no joke, Norm Bates. Norm and Merilyn Nance, my first psychology teacher, got me started down my convoluted and integrative academic path. And a special mention goes to Diane Freund for believing in my ability to write and eventually getting me to believe in it too.

Also appropriate is a shout out to all five of the NAU Religious Studies faculty while I was there: Bruce Sullivan, Peter van der Loo, Arne Massing, Sandra Lubarsky, and Wayne Mahan, for teaching me how to study ultimate questions.

Deepest respect to Macaela Cashman and Marcia Galleher, my first and always yoga teachers; to Gary Giangregorio, who taught me trataka and pranayama;

and to Georg Feuerstein, who continues to astound and inspire.

Nearly half of these teachers have passed on now, but I carry them with me in the person I am and the work I do.

All this knowledge would be worthless in a bubble. And so I acknowledge my close up and personal, everyday teachers: my parents, my siblings, my husband, and my son; the yoga teachers of Tucson who stop and ponder mysteries with me on the street; and the regulars who come to class and pretend to learn from me but really open themselves to their own wisdom.

Last but not least, I couldn't have done this on my own. Namaste to my co-creators: Tamara Lee Standard, whose inspiration and encouragement convinced me I could write this book in the first place; Susie Lantz, who has been everything you could want in an editor— patient, kind, knowledgeable, encouraging, and demanding; and Eric York, whose illustrations liven up these pages, with whom it's been a treat to work after twenty-eight years of friendship.

Immense gratitude fills my heart for all of you.

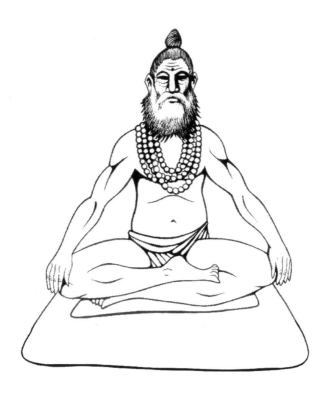

The Sadhu

INTRODUCTION:
THE STORY OF YOGA

Yoga is incredibly and increasingly popular. This is
because yoga is amazing. When most Americans hear
the word "yoga" they think of the stretches and postures
called *asana* (āsana) that come to us from Hatha Yoga,
and a well-rounded asana practice is indeed uniquely
healing. In fact it saved my life, which you can read all
about in my first book, *Yoga to Ease Anxiety*.

While most people come to yoga for its well-
documented health benefits, they stay because it offers
something deeper, more meaningful than other kinds of
exercise, and that is the opportunity to heal emotionally,
mature psychologically, and grow spiritually. There is,
undeniably, an emphasis on the physical in American
yoga culture. Even when the philosophy is taught, it's
usually from the perspect-ive of how we can apply it to
our lives today. This approach is super useful, but the
teachings themselves are often taken out of context,

which can lead to some confusion. What I hope to offer with this book is an introduction to the story of yoga, its history, and its philosophy in a linear way that is accessible to contemporary teachers and students of yoga.

It is not my intention to tell anyone what they have to believe or what they should or should not do in order to be a **yogi** or **yogini** (yoginī). I just want to relate the history of yoga and yogic ideas in a casual, relevant way.

It's taken me a long time to feel like I know enough to share this information. I first became interested in Eastern philosophies as a teenager after reading the Transcendentalists and Beat poets. As an undergrad, I was a Religious Studies major in a department that took a historical approach, and as a grad student I studied mysticism.

When I decided I was going to commit to the practice of yoga, I read everything about it I could find. And when I decided to do a 200-hour teacher training, I simultaneously enrolled in an 800-hour course in the History, Philosophy, and Literature of Yoga with the great yogic scholar Georg Feuerstein. I felt that if I were going to represent the tradition, I'd better understand it.

When yoga began, it was taught from one teacher to one student, both of whom had renounced the world in pursuit of spiritual liberation. I've been fascinated by the question of how yoga went from that intimate and dedicated scenario to hour-long classes at the local Y. As a teacher, I have continued to bump up against questions, situations in modern yoga that make no sense when compared to its austere history. So I kept reading,

2

researching, and trying to find answers. I've also spent the last few years serving as faculty for teacher trainings, where students often come up with some of the toughest and most interesting questions. Now I believe I have enough of the puzzle together to share it with others.

It's important to me to present an accurate picture of the yoga tradition. It's also important to me to present the information in a way that is relatable. Every topic of every chapter in this book has dozens of other books written just about it. And every single page here could be extended to its own chapter. That's how it goes with yoga: its history is so vast and compelling that when you walk through one door you enter another room full of doors. I make no claim to being comprehensive; that would be impossible.

I also make no claim to objectivity. This is the product of my investigation into the spiritual path I practice and teach. I weave the history of asana throughout the book because it's of interest to American yoga. And the texts I examine are the ones American yoga culture deems important. The translations I use are those that are accessible, as in both easily acquired and easily understood, or at least easier to understand than some of the more academically oriented translations.

My intentions and hopes are to provide a general history, to relate the fundamental philosophies of the yoga tradition, to tell the story of how yoga became what it is and made its way to America, and to spark interest and further investigation into this awesome, kaleidoscopic subject.

Our Map

The history of yoga gets wily in spots. In the beginning there are long stretches of homogeneity and then there are flurries of new ideas and cultural experiments. In the last three hundred years, yoga has been shaped in part by cross-cultural influences and interconnections. And more recently, dozens of individual personalities have grafted their own particular styles onto the tree of yoga.

To better organize our journey, we'll need a map. What follows is one of several possible approaches to categorizing the main events in the history of yoga. I find it to be the one that makes the story the most intelligible.

Pre-Vedic Age (7500 – 4500 BCE)[1, 2]: In the first chapter, "Ancient Mysticism and Asceticism," we'll talk about yoga's possible roots in shamanism and the prehistoric era of the Indus Valley civilization.

Vedic Age (4500 – 1500 BCE): The Vedas are the sacred scriptures that provide the foundation of all Hindu culture. Still in chapter 1, we'll look at the four Vedas for their spiritual and philosophical ideas in general and for early signs of yoga.

Upanishadic Age (1500 – 1000 BCE): In chapter 2, "The Forest Dwellers," we will encounter the *sannyasin*, or spiritual mendicant, and the beginnings of nondual philosophy. The Upanishads are early texts that provide the ideological roots of yoga.

Epic Age (1000 – 100 BCE): In "Great Warriors and the Age of Epics," we'll enter the stories of larger-than-life heroes and avatars. We'll examine the two illustrious epics of India, the *Ramayana* and the *Mahabharata*, for their contributions to yoga. Chapter 3 also contains a discussion of the *Bhagavad Gita*, which is one chapter in the *Mahabharata* and the first intentionally yogic text.

Classical Age (100 BCE – 500 CE): In chapter 4 we check out Patanjali's *Yoga Sutras*, learning about the philosophy behind Kriya Yoga and the eight limbs of Ashtanga. And in chapter 5 we find that the Upanishads continue to be influential as Shankara updates and propagates the Vedantic school of thought.

Tantric Age (500 – 1300 CE): Tantra represents a radical development in the history of yoga, democratizing spiritual growth for the masses. In chapter 6, "The Tantric Embrace of Reality," we'll explore both the origins of Tantra and its ideas about the energy body. Then in chapter 7 we look in on "The Yoga of the Body" through the classical texts of Hatha Yoga.

Empiric Age (1300 – 1800 CE): In chapter 8, "The Impact of Empires," we explore developments within yoga and Vedanta in the time of the Mughals, the East India Company, and the British Raj, all the way up to the first American encounters with yogic philosophy.

Modern Age (1800 – Present): In chapters 9 and 10 we come to understand the transition to modern postural yoga[3] and watch yoga make its way to the U.S. And in chapter 11 we witness the proliferation of "American Yoga" in the second half of the 20th century.

Because this is a book about the history of yoga, we will pay a lot more attention to the past than to the present. While we'll take a minute at the end to look at the issues and potential of modern-day American yoga, only time will give us the perspective to tell what trends will have a lasting influence.

Throughout the book, we will be covering more horizontal ground than vertical. That is to say, we won't be diving very deep into any one subject. Again, my intention is to provide an overview, an understanding of the big picture of yoga, and hopefully pique your interest in delving further into one area or another.

Along the way, we just might find that there is both a lot more and a lot less that historically falls under the umbrella of yoga than what is represented as doing so today. To show respect for the tradition and to avoid cultural misappropriation means first knowing what is and is not original to it.

Furthermore, for practitioners, having a clear understanding of yoga's history helps us to see our own experiences in context. As Feuerstein put it, "To learn about the historical evolution of Yoga is more than an academic exercise; it actually furthers our self-understanding and hence our efforts to swim free of the boundaries of the ego-personality."[4]

A Word about Words

Yoga comes to us from Sanskrit, which is the sacred language of the Hindu tradition. Sanskrit is an ancient language that derives from the same Indo-European family of languages as English, which is why we come across cognates every once in a while. "Yoga" is one of them. It means the same as the English word "yoke."

There's a lot of Sanskrit in this book. The first time we see a new Sanskrit word (and sometimes the second if they are far apart from one another) it will be italicized. And the first time we see a word that's in the glossary it will be in bold. There are a lot of words that are both.

At the moment, there are a few different standards for expressing Sanskrit words in English. One is to use the International Alphabet of Sanskrit Transliteration (IAST), which has lots of diacritical marks—lines and dots and tildes—on letters to signify how a letter should sound and which syllables should be emphasized. IAST is informative if you know what you're looking at, but not everybody does.

Another option is to give it our best go using just the plain old Roman alphabet. My compromise between ease of reading and wanting to be as accurate as possible is to list them both, if they are different, on the first usage of the word. I've put the IAST version in parentheses, as I've already done with (āsana) and (yoginī) above. After that, I use just the naked letters.

I would absolutely recommend spending some time with an online pronunciation guide with audio to learn how the words are supposed to sound. I like the one yoga teacher Tilak Pyle provides,[5] but you may find something that suits you better.

Yoga, Defined

Before we get much further, it's pretty important to define some terms, starting with the central idea of this entire project: yoga. We all have some sense of what we mean by yoga, but let's look at the historical development of its definition.

As we just saw, in straight translation "yoga" means "yoke," as in harnessing animals together, such as yoking horses together to pull a cart. This original meaning has been gently extended over time from "yoke" to "unite" to "union." You might have heard that "yoga" means "uniting" body and mind, left and right, sun and moon, higher and lower, and/or self and Self. This is where that definition comes from. Hopefully, by the end of this book all of those united pairs will make sense!

In the earliest sacred texts of India, the Vedas, "yoga" is most often used in this sense of yoking but other times means "discipline." This is discipline as in spiritual disciplines and austerities. Another word used in the Vedas to convey the same idea is *tapas*, which

8

means "heat" and refers to **ascetic** practices that build inner energy. Both yoga and tapas are used to signify the heat-building hard work of spiritual discipline: long meditations, fasting, penances, and so on.

The Upanishads are the next set of important texts in the yoga tradition. In them we start to see the word yoga used in a more **esoteric** way, meant to be interpreted or understood by those with special knowledge passed along from teacher to student. For instance, in the *Katha Upanishad* we find this:

When the senses are firmly reigned in,
that is Yoga, so people think.
From distractions a man is then free,
for Yoga is the coming-into-being,
as well as the ceasing-to-be.[6]

To break this down a little, yoga is first used here in the sense of withdrawing from the outside world ("senses firmly reigned in," free "from distractions"). Then it is defined as the "coming-into-being" and the "ceasing-to-be," which may mean that yoga is both the practice of unitive consciousness (being) and the disappearance of the ego in unitive consciousness (ceasing to be). Yoga is the discipline and the result of the discipline.

Next we arrive at the time of the epics and *Bhagavad Gita*, where the definition of yoga has expanded to encompass the many mystical paths of the Indian subcontinent. A mystical path is a course of action that leads to a direct experience of the Sacred. And this is one definition of yoga that we will keep returning to: yoga is the activity of seeking a direct experience of the Sacred.

Why Practice Yoga?

While we're defining terms, what is **Hinduism** exactly, and how is it different from yoga? Hinduism refers to the many religious and cultural traditions of India that trace their lineage back through the *Bhagavad Gita*, the Upanishads, and the Vedas. Hinduism is a broader category than yoga. Yoga is, or at least started as, one aspect of Hinduism—the part that provides techniques leading to ultimate spiritual liberation, freedom, or enlightenment. Other traditions that began in India, like Buddhism and Jainism, also developed their own yogic paths. In every case, the goal of yoga is the same: liberation.

Okay, but liberation from what? Freedom from what? Well, from suffering. We will talk a lot more about this as we go, but for now it's important to know that in the Hindu worldview, we are all in a continuous cycle of birth, life, death, and rebirth. This cycle is called *samsara* (saṁsāra). And this wheel of existence is fraught with sorrow for two interrelated reasons: ignorance and impermanence. Ignorance because we fundamentally misunderstand the truth of our reality, which is that the Sacred is the only eternal substance, making it the only thing that is ultimately real. And impermanence because we cling to the people and stuff of this world as if they were permanent and eternal, as if

10

they were real, when they are actually temporary and ephemeral. As long as we are ignorant of the truth about reality and remain attached to the material world, we keep coming back, being reborn, and enduring suffering.

We are stuck on this existential Ferris wheel, stuck in misunderstanding and reacting to the temporary as if it were eternal, because of two strong forces: *samskara* (saṃskāra) and *karma*. Samskara are deeply entrenched, tenacious habits of thought and action that are both innate and collect over time. And karma refers to actions and the consequences of our actions. The positive and negative effects of our actions pile up for and against us on a kind of cosmic abacus. Liberation means freedom from the cycle of samsara. It comes from burning through our karma with spiritual discipline and deconstructing our samskara by experiencing the Sacred first hand.

We don't have to believe in reincarnation to practice yoga. In Hinduism, the idea is that one lifetime is not enough to attain spiritual perfection. However, if reincarnation is a concept that doesn't sit easily with you, these ideas can still be helpful. The goal of yogic practices is to free ourselves from the good and bad results of our earlier decisions, to deconstruct our habits of thought and action, and to liberate our perspective from our encultured worldview. When we can see beyond our conditioning, we will see the world as it really is, Sacred.

To sum up the problem for which yoga is the solution, human life is full of suffering. We suffer because we don't understand the truth, which is that only the Sacred is eternal and real. Therefore we become attached to and misguided by what is impermanent. We get wrapped up in our temporary little dramas. And as long as we remain ignorant, our karma reinforces our samskara and keeps us in samsara. That is to say, our actions reinforce our habits and keep us in unenlightened existence.

The Paths of Yoga

Luckily, yoga provides many paths to spiritual liberation. In the next few sections of this chapter, we will look at some of the principal forms of yoga: Jnana, Bhakti, Karma, Tantra, and Hatha. These are by no means the only yogas, nor are they mutually exclusive. It's possible and even pretty standard for a person to blend two or more of them into their *sadhana* (sādhana) or yogic practice.

We will look at three components of each path: **metaphysics**, practices, and ultimate goal. By metaphysics I don't mean the kind of stuff you find in the psychic section of the bookstore. In philosophy, metaphysics refers to the study of what *is*. Metaphysics is how people answer the question, "What is the nature of reality?" And by practices I mean the actions one performs to instigate psycho-spiritual changes. Practices can include mental, emotional, and physical acts. And while each yoga has the same ultimate goal of spiritual freedom, this can be and is expressed in different ways. What follows is only a brief introduction to these concepts, beginning definitions to take with us on our adventure. We will come back and flesh out all of these ideas as we travel through the story of yoga.

Jnana Yoga

Jnana (jñāna) (pronounced *gyaana*) means "wisdom" or "knowledge." It's a cognate with the English word "gnosis," which means "mystical knowledge." The path of **Jnana Yoga** has a nondual metaphysics, which means it holds that all of reality is made out of one substance, not two or more. This **nondualism** is present in the Vedas and in the Upanishads, where we hear that there is only **Brahman**—the capital "R" Really Real and eternal sacred substance that has always existed and that created everything out of itself. Brahman is consciousness and the energy of creation. In Jnana Yoga, everything that is not the eternal Sacred is considered to be an illusion.

The central practices of Jnana Yoga are meditation, study, and renunciation. Renunciation means giving up *everything*—occupation, family, material goods, and even one's name. Getting rid of these distractions helps the renunciate to focus on the difference between what is temporary and unreal and what is eternal and real. The goal of Jnana Yoga is, first, to have a direct experience of the Sacred, and second, to live with that experience always in mind, thereby gaining distance and freedom from the sufferings of the illusory world.

Bhakti Yoga

Bhakti Yoga is the path of divine love. It is the theistic tradition of devotion to an individual's chosen and cherished deity, called an *ishta devata* (iṣṭadevatā).

13

Bhakti metaphysics can range from **qualified non-dualism** to **dualism**. In qualified nondualism there is only the supreme deity, whatever he or she is called. It's nondual because there is only the deity, but qualified because the deity is greater than the created universe. In other words, the deity created the world out of its own substance but exists beyond the world as well. A dualist bhakti metaphysics holds that the deity created the universe, but he or she is separate from creation.

The practices of Bhakti Yoga include contemplating and meditating on the divine form, *kirtan*-style chanting, ritual worship, and prostration. Grace is an important idea in Bhakti Yoga. While a *bhakta* strives to maintain an attitude of constant sacrifice and self-offering, it is only through the grace of their ishta devata that a person can merge with the divine and be free of samsara and suffering. Because a person does not have to renounce the world to practice Bhakti Yoga, it is a common choice for householders.

Karma Yoga

Karma Yoga is the yoga of self-transcending action. According to this path, we all must live according to our *dharma* or duty. Originally, dharma signified both living in accord with *rita* (ṛta), which is the principle of cosmic order, and doing the work appropriate to our station in life, which for millennia meant sticking to your **caste**. We will see as we travel through the history of yoga that caste has played a very large role.

To practice Karma Yoga is to perform all actions in the spirit of inner sacrifice and without being attached to the outcome of our actions. When this attitude is perfected, we no longer acquire new karma and we become free from samsara. Karma Yoga is often practiced alongside Bhakti, as a way to stay in the world yet still transcend it.

Tantra Yoga

Tantra translates as "loom" or "web." Emerging in the centuries around the turn of the first millennium, **Tantra Yoga** claims to be a path for our current degenerate age, called the **Kali Yuga**. Metaphysically, it follows the Upanishads and Jnana Yoga in being nondual and claiming that "All is One." Where it differs is in emphasizing that, if All is One, then the material world is also a manifestation of the Sacred. For Tantra, nothing exists that is not divine. Everything and everyone is Sacred, regardless of caste or gender, regardless of social rules and taboos.

Tantric practices include *mantra* (repetition of sacred sounds), *mudra* (energy seals performed with the whole body or just the hands), *yantras* and *mandalas* (symbolic diagrams), and rituals—lots of rituals. Many *tantrikas*, people who practice Tantra Yoga, are devotees of the goddess **Shakti** (Śakti), who represents the feminine, creative form of the Sacred. The deity **Shiva** (Śiva) is her partner and mate. He represents pure consciousness.

New with Tantra Yoga and central to its offspring **Hatha Yoga** is the importance of the **subtle body**. Also called the energy body, the subtle body is made up of *prana* (life energy, like *chi* in Chinese medicine) flowing through **nadis** or channels. The spinal column holds pride of place in this configuration, marking the location of the most important nadi, the **sushumna** (suṣumṇa). In most of us, this channel is blocked by Shakti, in her form as the **kundalini**, lying coiled and dormant at the base of the spine. Liberation occurs when our kundalini awakens and flows freely through this central channel, connecting with the Shiva energy at the crown of the head.

Hatha Yoga

Hatha translates as "force," and the metaphysics of Hatha Yoga is the same as in Tantra, nondualism—All is One. Hatha Yoga came from the **Siddha** (perfected) Movement within Tantra. Tantra was already saying everything in the material world is sacred; the siddhas shifted the focus to the body.

Building on the foundation laid by previous types of yoga, Hatha Yoga espouses both physical and mental practices. On the physical side there are purification rituals called the **shat karma** (ṣaṭ-karman) as well as asana, mudra, and **bandha**, which are energy locks. Spanning the physical and the mental are **pratyahara** (pratyāhāra), which is the practice of sense withdrawal, and **pranayama** (prāṇāyāma), which are breath control and extension exercises. Then there are **dhyana** (dhyāna), which refers to being absorbed in meditation, and **samadhi** (samādhi) also known as union, both of which are purely states of consciousness. Hatha yogis view their approach as more complete than other paths because it includes the entire body-mind. Liberation for

Hatha Yoga is the same as in Tantra, and includes clearing the energy body of the seeds of karma and moving the kundalini up the sushumna.

Concluding the Introduction

Yoga provides different paths for different temperaments and stages of life. It has collected these elements over its very long history, never discarding a previous practice or belief but always simply adding to its repertoire of means of approaching the Sacred. Outfitted with this general information, we now head into the distant past to trace the threads that weave the web of yoga.

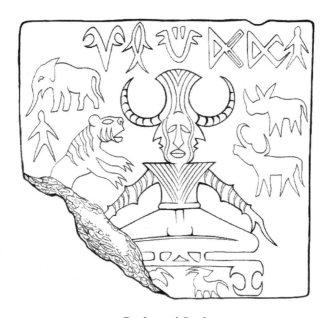

Pashupati Seal

1 ANCIENT MYSTICISM AND ASCETICISM

Now, the story of yoga. Most accounts of yoga's past begin by examining the longest continuously revered set of texts in human history, the Vedas, and we will indeed spend a good part of this chapter on Vedic beliefs and practices. But before we get to the Vedas, we need to make a stop at the Indus Valley civilization. And even before we get to the Indus Valley, to go as far back as we can possibly go, we will visit the shamans.

Yoga and Shamanism

Shamans are the gate keepers to the spiritual realm for tribal societies. Mircea Eliade, a primary figure in the academic study of yoga, was also one of the first to seriously inquire into shamanism. He called the practices of this global phenomenon "techniques of ecstasy."[1] Shamans hold a magical view of life, and their beliefs and practices have much in common with those of yoga. We don't know if these similarities are due to yoga having roots in shamanism or are just fascinating coincidences, but similarities do abound.

Both shamans and yogis hold the soul to be a type of energy body that is usually coextensive with the physical body but can detach and travel on its own. This subtle body participates in out-of-body experiences like magical flight, bilocation, and transmigration, during which the soul enters and can control another being.

Shamans and yogis also use similar methods to induce altered states of consciousness, including chanting, drumming, and psychotropic drugs. For yogis, in the early days this drug was a drink called *soma*, possibly made with the hallucinogenic mushroom fly agaric (*amanita muscaria*), and over the last several hundred years many yogis have used marijuana in the form of *bhang* or *ganja*. Yogis and shamans are also both known as healers and mind readers. Both groups submit themselves to intense austerities and trials, and both participate in symbolic death experiences.

As we move through the story of yoga, these similarities will continue to crop up. But for now, archeologists don't have any hard evidence of a direct link between shamanism and yoga. It's all just intriguing speculation.

The Indus Valley Civilization

Moving on to the still prehistoric Indus Valley civilization, we find the largest structured society of the ancient world. Situated in what is now Pakistan and northwest India, in the lands surrounding the Indus and Sarasvati rivers, this society covered nearly five hundred thousand square miles, which is almost double the size of Texas. Incredibly advanced for its time, the Indus Valley's large cities were planned around granaries and citadels; its houses had indoor bathrooms that fed into covered sewers; and there is even evidence of trade with places as far away as central Asia and Crete.[2]

Despite everything that archeologists have discovered about the Indus Valley culture, there's even more that they haven't. Only tens of some two thousand potential locations have been excavated, in part due to the logistical problems of sites being buried under dozens of feet of mud. Even among those digs archeologists have been able to start, some have stalled out due to permanent flooding.

Two facts archeologists have been able to determine are that (1) the oldest city yet unearthed dates to around 6500 BCE or earlier and (2) the Sarasvati River dried up over a number of years and was gone by around 1900 BCE.

Until the Vedas, there isn't a lot to go by to tell what the religious beliefs of this civilization entailed. All we have are several soapstone seals, which may have been stamps merchants used to mark their goods. These seals feature pictures that bear a striking resemblance to both early Vedic symbolism and later Hindu motifs. One seal in particular has caught the imagination of people who study yoga.

The illustration at the beginning of this chapter is of the Pashupati Seal. Pashupati means "Lord of the Animals," and we see here a horned man or maybe deity, surrounded by what scholars figure to be a rhinoceros and a buffalo on the upper right, an elephant and a tiger on the left, and antelope beneath.

Many have seen consistencies between this figure and Shiva, the Lord of Yoga. In later eras, one of Shiva's many epithets will be Pashupati, and some scholars have seen enough resemblance in the figure's seated position, dispassionate appearance, and animal entourage to postulate that he is a kind of proto-Shiva. It is also possible to make out an erection, though some interpret these markings as tassels hanging from the figure's waist. If it was intended as more phallic than finery, it would further tie this symbol with Shiva. Erections are a symbol of creative power and controlled energy. Shiva is well-known for his.

Again, as with shamanism, it's all speculation. It's just a picture with no commentary. Perhaps if someone figures out how to decipher the symbols at the top of the seal, we'll have a better idea of what is represented here. For now, we have to wait until the Vedas, which came at least two thousand years after the Indus Valley civilization began, to know anything for certain about what they believed.

Dating the Vedas

The bedrock of Indian culture is formed by the four books collectively called the Vedas. The Vedas are seriously old; however, assigning a date to their origin is tricky. In the main, this is because the texts were passed down orally through certain families of the **brahmin** (priestly) class. This makes eminent sense in a tropical location where the very weather is hostile toward paper and in a culture that was repeatedly invaded. The safest place to keep a text was inside people. However, for us it means there is unlikely to be any physical evidence to help establish a date.

We do know that the earliest parts of the Vedas originated while the Sarasvati River still flowed, since the goddess Sarasvati plays a very important role as a sort of patron saint of the entire civilization. With the combined expertise of archeologists and linguists, the best guess at this point is that the Vedas attained their current form sometime between 4500 and 2500 BCE. To put it more generally, the Vedas are about five thousand years old.

The Four Books

Early Vedic culture was based on ritual sacrifices to appease deities and maintain the order of the universe. The four Vedas, the *Rig Veda*, the *Sama Veda,* the *Yajur Veda,* and the *Atharva Veda*, were the texts that they relied on to do it correctly. Let's look at each in turn.

Rig Veda (Ṛg Veda): "Veda" means "knowledge" or "wisdom" and "rig" (or ṛg) means "praise," so the *Rig Veda* is the "Knowledge of Praise." It is the oldest and longest of the Vedas, and long it is at around 10,600 verses in 1,028 hymns. Most of the hymns are invocations and prayers to deities, although there are also mythological stories and accounts of the creation of the world.

Sama Veda (Sāma Veda): This book's name translates into "Knowledge of Songs." It contains the verses that are chanted during sacrificial rituals. Most of these (1,800 of 1,875) are from the *Rig Veda.* The centrality of chanting in early Vedic religion probably led to an interest in the effect of patterned breathing and from there to pranayama.

Yajur Veda: The *Yajur Veda,* "Knowledge of Sacrifice," contains the hymns necessary for sacrificial rituals. Again, it contains mostly verses that originally appear in the *Rig Veda.*

Atharva Veda: Finally, the *Atharva Veda* was admitted to the canon much later than the first three. It was named after the great seer, or **rishi,** Atharvan. This volume contains many magical incantations for healing, protection, and wealth, as well as more metaphysical passages, such as philosophical riddles and speculations about prana and pranayama.

As previously mentioned, the overwhelming emphasis of the Vedas is sacrificial ritual to maintain cosmic order. There are sacrifices designed for both brahmins and householders. Besides supplications and prayers, the Vedas also contain creation myths and insights into different social groups in Vedic culture. It is important as we skim the surface of what the Vedas have to say to remember that the Vedic religion is still alive today. In fact, it is the oldest continuously practiced religion in the world.

Creation

Creation myths from around the world tell of the origin of all things. They are usually "cosmogonical," meaning that they describe how order came out of chaos at the beginning of time. There are several creation myths in the Vedas. We will look at two that characterize the philosophical and reverent demeanor of the Vedas, respectively.

The first takes a pragmatic view of creation and is not hesitant to admit what we cannot know. Its topics are the inscrutable nature of what existed before creation and the fundamental qualities of tapas (heat, austerities) and *kama* (love, desire).

At first was neither Being nor Nonbeing.
There was not air nor yet sky beyond.
What was its wrapping? Where? In whose
     protection?
Was Water there, unfathomable and deep?

There was no death then, nor yet deathlessness;
of night or day there was not any sign.
The One breathed without breath, by its own
     impulse.

25

Other than that was nothing else at all.

Darkness was there, all wrapped around by darkness,
and all was Water indiscriminate. Then
that which was hidden by the Void, that One,
    emerging,
stirring, through power of Ardor (tapas), came to be.

In the beginning Love (kama) arose,
which was the primal germ cell of the mind.
The Seers, searching in their hearts with wisdom,
discovered the connection of Being in Nonbeing.

A crosswise line cut Being from Nonbeing.
What was described above it, what below?
Bearers of seed there were and mighty forces,
thrust from below and forward move above.

Who really knows? Who can presume to tell it?
When was it born? Whence issued the creation?
Even the Gods came after its emergence.
Then who can tell from whence it came to be?

That out of which creation has arisen,
whether it held it firm or it did not,
He who surveys it in the highest heaven,
He surely knows—or maybe He knows not![3]

This passage is simultaneously beautiful and difficult. On the surface we've been told that first there was neither Being nor Nonbeing. Then the One emerged due to tapas, or its own internally generated heat, and created the world from the seed of kama, desire. Many passages in the Vedas are written in this heavily symbolic and esoteric style. Some scholars have posited that there must have been a code that is now lost, some sort of cypher with which to solve the riddles. Some mystics say that with right understanding the truth of the Vedas reveals itself.

"The One" is a stunningly abstract concept that deserves special notice. Here is a five-thousand-year-old idea claiming that all that exists comes from a singularity. The One lays the foundation for the nondualism followed by most branches of yoga philosophy.

Our next creation story turns to the gods and foreshadows the devotional direction of yoga and the interconnection between religion and social structures. In it we watch the gods sacrifice ***Purusha*** (cosmic man). From Purusha come the ***varnas*** (the major classes or castes of Hindu society), the sun and moon, and the elemental deities.

> When they divided up the Man,
> Into how many parts did they divide him?
> What did his mouth become: What his arms?
> What are his legs called? What his feet?
>
> His mouth became the brahmin; his arms
> became the warrior-prince, his legs
> the common man who plies his trade.
> The lowly serf was born from his feet.
> The Moon was born from his mind; the Sun

came into being from his eye;
from his mouth came Indra and Agni,
while from his breath the Wind was born.
With the sacrifice the Gods sacrificed to the
    sacrifice.
Those were the first established rites.
These powers ascended up to heaven
where dwell the ancient gods and other beings.[4]

Besides illustrating the creative power of the gods, we see here how deeply rooted the caste system was in Indian tradition, with the four main varnas delineated in the oldest of texts. Those four castes are the brahmins or priests, the *kshatriya* or warriors, the *vaishya* or merchants, and the *shudra* (śūdra) or servant class. Even below the shudra were the outcastes, the **untouchables**. The caste system shaped the Indian experience for millennia before it was constitutionally abolished in 1950.

Gods and Goddesses

Since, in the Vedic worldview, creation began with the gods making a sacrifice, it followed that sacrifice was meaningful to the gods and would gain their attention and hopefully their favor. By far, the majority of Vedic verses are supplications to deities. The most mentioned gods are Indra, god of thunder; Agni, god of fire; and Soma, god of the intoxicating soma drink. Important goddesses are Vac, goddess of speech; Ushas, goddess of dawn; and Sarasvati, the deification of the great river.

An important if lesser Vedic deity is Rudra, the Howler. Rudra was the wild, unpredictable god of storms and of the hunt. Later he will merge with Shiva, Lord of Yoga.

Though there are said to be 3,339 deities, only 33 are mentioned by name. And, as we see in the following verse, all of the deities are part of the One.

> They call him Indra, Mitra, Varuna,
> Agni or the heavenly sunbird Garumat.
> The Seers call in many ways that which is One;
> they speak of Agni, Yama, Mātariśvan.[5]

Again, this is pretty incredible. Here in the first book of the oldest collection of sacred books in the world, we see an integration of polytheism and monotheism. From the beginning, all the many gods and goddesses of India have been recognized as different faces of the One, an all-encompassing, ultimate Sacred Being.

Rishis, Keshins, and Vratyas

There are three groups of mystics referred to in the Vedas. They are, in all likelihood, the forerunners of the yogic tradition. These groups are the rishis, the *keshins*, and the *vratyas* (vrātyas).

While most of the Vedic ceremonies are sacrificial rituals performed by brahmins, the Vedas were not written by brahmins but by rishis. Through contemplation and austerities, the ancient rishis made contact with the One, and they came back with the verses of the Vedas.

(The Vedas, therefore, are considered **shruti**, which means "that which was heard," indicating they are the direct transliteration of the Sacred. Other shruti texts are the *Brahmanas [Brāhmanas]* and the *Aranyakas*, which will be described later in this chapter, and the Upanishads, which we cover in the next chapter. Sacred texts that don't fall under shruti are considered **smriti**, "that which was remembered.") Besides being discovered in mystical trance states, at least some of the Vedic hymns are the result of competitions held between members of brotherhoods of rishis.

Unlike the rishis, the keshins and vratyas were not accepted as part of Vedic culture. The keshins, or long-haired ascetics, apparently lived on the fringes of society. This group is described in the following verses from the *Rig Veda*.

Within him is fire, within him is drink,
within him both earth and heaven.
He is the Sun which views the whole world,
he is indeed light itself—
the long-haired ascetic.

Girded with the wind, they have donned ocher mud
for a garment. So soon as the Gods
have entered within them, they follow the wings
of the wind, these silent ascetics.

Intoxicated, they say, by our austerities,
we have taken the winds for our steeds.

You ordinary mortals here below
see nothing except our bodies.

He flies through midair, the silent ascetic,
beholding the forms of all things.
To every God he has made himself
a friend and collaborator.

Ridden by the wind, companion of its blowing,
pushed along by the Gods,
he is at home in both seas, the East
and the West—this silent ascetic.

He follows the track of all the spirits,
of nymphs and the deer of the forest.
Understanding their thoughts, bubbling
      with ecstasies,
their appealing friend is he—
the long-haired ascetic.

The wind has prepared and mixed him a drink;
it is pressed by Kunamnamā.
Together with Rudra he has drunk from the cup
of poison—the long-haired ascetic.[6]

This is a phenomenal passage, tying the keshins back to shamanism and possibly forward to tantric practices. It begins by describing the keshin as encompassing "both earth and heaven" and more. This is the mystical identity of union. "Girded with the wind" means naked, and "clothed in ocher mud" may have

31

been a preliminary practice to covering the body in ashes as yogis have done for millennia and continue to do today. Then there is a description of magical flight, linking the keshin to the shaman. That he "follows the track" of spirits, nymphs, and deer, "understanding their thoughts, bubbling with ecstasies" may be intended to again illustrate the mystic's oneness with all things, on all planes of existence. Kunamnama is the name of a dark-natured female deity who is mentioned only here and nowhere else in all the Vedas. She could foreshadow the tantric devotion to fierce forms of the feminine divine. And the word that is translated as "poison" can also be translated as "drug"—another indication that keshins experimented with ecstatic altered states of consciousness, again promoting the view of continuity between shamanism and yoga. Finally, they share their cup with the wild god Rudra, who becomes Shiva, the Lord of Yoga. Keshins, we can extrapolate, were spiritual bad asses.

The third group foreshadowing yoga is described in book 15 of the *Atharva Veda*, which is called the *Vratya Khanda*. Vratyas were nomads. They traveled in groups or alone and were so far outside the cultural boundaries of Vedic society that they were considered fit for sacrifice by brahmins and may have actually been used as such in the early, literal period of the Vedic religion.

There is little doubt that the vratyas were fore-runners of yoga. There are signs that they practiced pranayama; held a nondual philosophy; worshipped Rudra; used the sacred mantra Om; and that at least some of them were celibate—all of these are foundational elements of the yoga tradition. So, while we have adequate if cursory evidence to suggest these yogic elements existed, they remained culturally tangential until much later in our story. That is to say, the Vedic culture was the ruling power and these guys were outsiders, so these practices are rarely mentioned until much later, when many of these marginalized elements come together under the umbrella of Tantra Yoga.

The Lineage of the Vedas

In the end, the Vedas are a sprawling, inspirational wonder. They are the basis of the oldest living religious tradition, simultaneously an artifact and a way of life. The Vedas provide a fascinating window to the past and the foundation on which nearly all of Indian culture is built. There are several lifetimes worth of study here for those who are called to it. And for the rest of us, it is a beginning, a starting point in the story of yoga.

Eventually, over several generations, the rishis faded from the scene. The Vedas continued to be transmitted orally—memorized and recited by rote—and the priests continued to perform the sacrifices, but their understanding of the meaning behind the words they spoke declined. As the Sarasvati River dried up, what had been the Indus Valley culture moved east, toward the Ganges River basin.

New texts called the *Brahmanas* and *Aranyakas* came about to explain the dense symbolism of the Vedas. The *Brahmanas* are digests of the Vedas and pay special attention to proper performance of rituals.

"Aranyaka" means "of the forest," and these books explain the more powerful sacrifices, the idea being that these rituals are too dangerous to be spoken of in populated areas and should only be taught and practiced out in the forest, away from civilization. It is also possible that the *Aranyakas* mark a crossover between traditional Vedic brahmins and the lifestyle of the keshins and vratyas. That is to say, it may have been at this point that serious spiritual seekers from within the Vedic community started renouncing family and village life and heading to the forest to seek enlightenment.

If it wasn't at this point it was soon after, because that was the M.O. of the originators of the beautiful and mystical Upanishads, the subject of our next chapter.

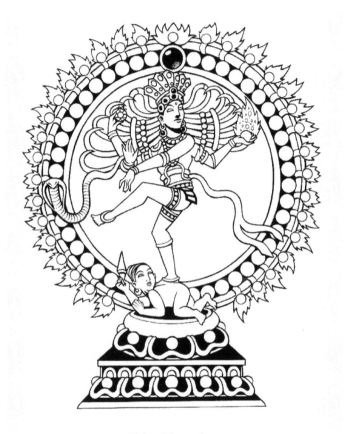

Shiva Nataraja

2 THE FOREST DWELLERS

The time is 2,500 years ago. The place is the Gangetic plain, a fertile land in what is now northeast India, bounded on the north by the imposing Himalayas. Our subjects are the forest dwellers, spiritual seekers who have abandoned familial and material comforts in their quest for enlightenment and liberation.

The search for meaning is innate to human nature, though some of us are more taken by it than others. In ancient India, those who could not ignore the great questions of life retreated to the wilderness and turned within to find answers. What they discovered was recorded in the Upanishads.

The Upanishads

This word, "upanishad," when taken apart means "to sit down near" or "to sit close to." That is how the stories and lessons of the Upanishads were originally communicated, with the student sitting down near the teacher. But in context, within the stories and lessons themselves, the word "upanishad" means something more like "secret teaching" or "hidden connection."

To be granted this hidden knowledge of the forest dwellers, one first had to become a sannyasin, a renunciate. We saw in the previous chapter that renunciation was not unknown in ancient India. Keshins and vratyas were early examples of forgoing the niceties of civilization in order to concentrate on the life of the spirit. Over time, the idea that a person had to give up everything to find enlightenment became deeply entrenched in Indian culture. And while walking away from everything has never been the mainstream thing to do, it did get to the point where some rules had to be laid down.

The span of a spiritual man's life came to be divided into four stages: student, householder, forest dweller, and sannyasin.[1] In the forest-dwelling stage, which could begin only after one's first grandchild was born, it was not necessary to take sannyasa. A man could live near his village and even have his wife with him. In the final stage, he would renounce everything and become a wandering mendicant. Of course, there have always been those who skip the middle two stages and go straight from student to sannyasin.

Renouncing, however, was just the first step. Next came finding a guru, a trusted guide to the spiritual realm. And eventually, when the guru judged the seeker as worthy, only then would the secret wisdom be shared.

In this way, the contents of the Upanishads were transmitted orally, one-on-one, from teacher to student through generations. And while the material is pretty esoteric in places, the meaning behind the words would have been explained and ruminated upon in this guru-disciple relationship.

Unlike the keshins and the vratyas who were considered outcastes, the people who composed the Upanishads were well within the Vedic tradition. In many ways the lessons of the Upanishads represent a refinement of the spiritual teachings of the Vedas, including the mystical internalization of the ritual sacrifice.

There are several Upanishads. Because 108 is a sacred number in Hinduism, there are said to be 108 Upanishads; however, there are over 200 in existence. Different sects leave out and include various texts to make the numbers add up. The early Upanishads, of which there are around a dozen, are called *mukhya*, meaning "chief." Some of these originated as part of the *Brahmanas* and *Aranyakas*, around the 7th to 5th centuries BCE, and the rest were composed between then and the beginning of the Common Era. Later Upanishads come from between the beginning of the Common Era until the Middle Ages. For the most part, what we cover will be from the mukhya Upanishads.

The Upanishads are not in any way systematized. Each one is a collection of verses, sayings, stories, and lessons passed down from and about ancient sages. My intentions here are threefold: (1) to explain the main philosophical concepts of the Upanishads, (2) to introduce some of the segments that are the most influential today, and (3) to, when possible, let them speak in their own bafflingly beautiful words.

Big Ideas

To begin to understand the significance of the Upanishads, we must first establish a lexicon. There are five intertwining ideas that are central to the philosophy of these texts; they are *Brahman*, *atman*, *samsara*, *karma*, and *moksha*. Some of these terms have already been defined in the Introduction. Because these concepts are so important to our story, we need to take the time to get more familiar with them and understand how they are related to one another. We'll do this briefly here and in more depth throughout the rest of the chapter.

Brahman: The Vedas had already made it clear that (1) creation came about through the will of the One, and that (2) though gods and goddesses are called by many names, really there is only the One. In the Upanishads, the One is called Brahman. As we saw in the Introduction, Brahman is the Ultimate Reality and creative principle. It is genderless, all pervasive, infinite, and eternal. It is truth and bliss. Brahman does not change but is the cause of all change. It is both immanent (within all things) and transcendent (above all things). It is the binding unity of creation. Many translate Brahman as the ground of being or God.

Atman: This is the soul. <u>Each of us has an ***atman***</u> (ātman), an individual soul that is our true Self. This is not the ego personality. Our personalities are changeable and temporary. The atman is that part of us that is eternal and unchanging, and it is identical with Brahman. Our essential being is exactly the same as the sacred essence of all that exists.

Samsara: But we get lost in the superficial world around us and forget that we are part of the Sacred. Our forgetfulness of our true nature keeps us trapped in samsara, the wheel of birth, life, death, and rebirth, the wheel of reincarnation. And this cycle of living and dying is stuffed to the gills with suffering. In our ignorance, we give the changeable, impermanent aspects of creation ultimate importance, and because we do we become attached to what is doomed to disappear, and we feel aversion toward those things that cause us discomfort.

Karma: As long as we persist in our habitually misguided ideas about what is ultimately real, we continue to accrue karmic debts. Karma refers to the consequences of our actions: bad or unwise actions lead to negative consequences, and good or wise actions lead to positive consequences. In relation to samsara, karma determines the conditions of our continued rebirths.

Moksha: The goal of spiritual discipline, according to the Upanishads, is to realize that atman is Brahman.

Not just to know it intellectually, but to experience the unity of all things and to live in the realization of that unity. When we are enlightened in this way, we see the true nature of all that is. We no longer acquire new karmic debts and our old karma is destroyed. Then, when we die, we merge with Brahman and we are liberated from samsara. This liberation is ***moksha*** (mokṣa).

To put all of these ideas together in one sentence: Karma keeps us stuck in samsara until we achieve moksha by experiencing the unity of atman and Brahman. Or, without the Sanskrit, our habits keep us stuck in a rut of suffering until we achieve enlightenment by realizing we are one with the Sacred.

Brahman and Atman

One of the most important philosophical foundations of the Upanishads is its metaphysical nondualism. Let's break that down. As we have seen, a system's "meta-physics" means how it sums up what is. In the philosophy of the Upanishads, the only thing that is really real is Brahman. Everything else, including you and I, was created by and is permeated by Brahman. So, it's nondual since it claims the world is made of only one substance. For comparison, modern Western philosophy, based on the metaphysics of Descartes and other Age of Reason thinkers, is a dualism consisting of two completely different substances: mind and matter. Brahman is both mind and matter, consciousness and energy.

In the *Brihadaranyaka Upanishad*, or *Great Hidden Teaching of the Forest*, we find the following descriptions of the ultimate nature of Brahman, and by extension atman, since atman is of the same substance as Brahman.

> In the beginning this world was only *brahman*, and it knew only itself (*ātman*), thinking: "I am *brahman*." As a result, it became the Whole. Among the gods, likewise, whosoever realized this, only they became the Whole. It was the same also among the seers and among humans.

> This *brahman* is without a before and an after, without an inner and an outer. *Brahman* is the self (*ātman*) here which perceives everything.

> As all the spokes are fastened to the hub and the rim of a wheel, so to one's self (*ātman*) are fastened all beings, all the gods, all the worlds, all the breaths, and all these bodies (*ātman*). [2]

It's not that we don't exist because only Brahman exists; it's that we are Brahman. And just like Brahman, we are everything. One way to envision it is that everything is interconnected in one big web and, because it's all the same substance, every part is also at the same time the web as a whole.

Later, when the teachings of the Upanishads are systematized by Vedanta, Brahman will be identified as energy and consciousness, which makes this a little easier to wrap our heads around. Follow me here: Since Brahman is consciousness as well as all the energy (and therefore matter) of the universe, all the different nodes on this great big web of existence can be seen as interconnecting points of consciousness. These points are able to see from their own perspectives, and through yogic disciplines, we can tap into the whole and see from any perspective or from all perspectives at once, because it is all fundamentally the same consciousness.

Mahavakyas

The ultimate nature of Brahman and our relation to Brahman through the atman are reiterated throughout the Upanishads, especially in the **mahavakyas** or great sayings. There are four original mahavakyas, and each one states some aspect of the message that flows throughout all of the texts. Here they are, in Sanskrit and in English:

~ *Prajñānam brahma*: Wisdom is Brahman.
~ *Ayam ātmā brahma*: Atman is Brahman.
~ *Tat tvam asi*: That art thou or you are That.
~ *Aham brahmāsmi*: I am Brahman.

One of these phrases is just a little more obscure than the others. While profound, "consciousness is Brahman," "atman is Brahman," and "I am Brahman," are fairly succinct given what we already know. "You are That," on the other hand, requires some explaining.

It comes from the story of Śvetaketu learning about Brahman and atman from his father, Uddālaka.

Shvetaketu has just returned from receiving his education, and not unlike a political science major home for the holidays, he thinks he knows way more than his dad now. That is, until Uddalaka asks if he's learned the rule of substitution.

"You seem to be proud of all this learning,"
Said Uddalaka. "But did you ask
Your teacher for that spiritual wisdom
Which enables you to hear the unheard,
Think the unthought, and know the unknown?"

Shvetaketu admits he hasn't learned anything like that. Uddalaka explains the rule of substitution by saying,

"As by knowing one lump of clay, dear one,
We come to know all things made out of clay
That they differ only in name and form,
While the stuff of which all are made is clay
. . . ."

And this rule, Uddalaka goes on to say, holds true for gold, for iron, and even for spirit. Uddalaka tells Shvetaketu that in the beginning there was "one without a second." That was Brahman, which is translated in the following as the Self. Brahman made all things out of itself, and "You are that, Shvetaketu; you are that." He goes on to explain Brahman's permeation of creation with various metaphors. (The beautiful translation I've been using here comes from Eknath Easwaran. The brackets represent my gender-neutral adaption of Easwaran's use of the masculine pronoun.)

"As bees suck nectar from many a flower
And make their honey one, so that no drop
Can say, 'I am from this flower or that,'
All creatures, though one, know not they are that
    One.
There is nothing that does not come from [it].
Of everything, [it] is the inmost Self. [It] is the truth;
[it] is the Self supreme.
You are that, Shvetaketu; you are that."

"As the rivers flowing east and west
Merge in the sea and become one with it,
Forgetting they were ever separate rivers,
So do all creatures lose their separateness
When they merge at last into pure Being.
There is nothing that does not come from [it].
Of everything, [it] is the inmost Self. [It] is the truth;
[it] is the Self supreme.
You are that, Shvetaketu; you are that."

"Please, Father, tell me more about this Self," asks Shvetaketu.

"Yes, dear one, I will," Uddalaka said.
"Place this salt in water and bring it here
Tomorrow morning." The boy did.
"Where is that salt?" his father asked.
"I do not see it."

46

"Sip here. How does it taste?"

"Salty, Father."

"And here? And there?"

"I taste salt everywhere."

"It *is* everywhere, though we see it not.

Just so, dear one, the Self is everywhere,

Within all things, although we see [it] not.

There is nothing that does not come from [it].

Of everything, [it] is the inmost Self. [It] is the truth;

    [it] is the Self supreme.

You are that, Shvetaketu; you are that."

And that is the meaning behind "Tat tvam asi"—You are That. Brahman so thoroughly permeates reality that to know one part is to know all by the rule of substitution. The section ends assuring us that Shvetaketu did indeed learn from his father:

"Then Shvetaketu understood this teaching

Truly, he understood it all."[3]

Reincarnation

According to the Upanishads, samsara is mostly the pits. In fact, the Upanishads base the need for liberation on the reality of reincarnation. Not only do we keep coming back and going around again and again, but depending on our karma we could come back not just as any caste or station in life but as any life form, from plant to insect to reptile and so on. A human birth, then, is super important. It is the only form in which we are self-conscious enough to ask the big, metaphysical questions about existence and seek after answers of a spiritual nature. It is a precious opportunity to break the cycle and escape from samsara.

So, where did the idea of reincarnation originate? In the Vedas there is one verse that hints at a soul returning and "wearing new life." And in the oldest Upanishad, the *Bhrihadaranyaka*, we find this:

> As a caterpillar, having come to the end of one blade of grass, draws itself together and reaches out for the next, so the Self, having come to the end of one life and dispelled all ignorance, gathers in [its] faculties and reaches out from the old body to a new.

The reason we keep coming back is to fulfill our unfinished karma, which will continue to accrue and play itself out until we learn to let go of our attachments. Then we become immortal—truly free to live forever in union with Brahman. To continue in the words of the *Brihadaranyaka Upanishad*, it sounds like this:

> As a person acts, so he becomes in life. Those who do good become good; those who do harm become bad. Good deeds make one pure; bad deeds make one impure. You are what your deep, driving desire is. As your desire is, so is your will. As your will is, so is your deed. As your deed is, so is your destiny.

We live in accordance with our deep driving desire. It is this desire at the time of death that determines

what our next life will be. We will come back to
earth to work out the satisfaction of that desire.

But not those who are free from desire; they are free
because all their desires have found fulfillment in the
Self. They do not die like the others; but realizing
Brahman, they merge in Brahman. So it is said:

When all the desires that surge in the heart
Are renounced, the mortal becomes immortal.
When all the knots that strangle the heart
Are loosened, the mortal becomes immortal.
Here in this very life. [4]

The idea of reincarnation could have any number of
sources. These days a common explanation is that we
have to keep coming back because one lifespan doesn't
give us enough time to achieve enlightenment. Some
people claim that the idea of reincarnation is just wishful
thinking, an attempt to deny the finality of death. But
that doesn't seem a likely starting point given the ani-
mosity most Upanishadic sages had toward this life,
which is nowhere stated with quite the same vehemence
as in the *Maitrayaniya Upanishad* (which is not counted
as one of the early Upanishads but was written before
the Common Era):

Venerable, in this ill-smelling, unsubstantial body
[which is nothing but] a conglomerate of bone, skin,
sinew, muscle, marrow, flesh, semen, blood, mucus,
tears, rheum, feces, urine, wind, bile, and phlegm—

what good is the enjoyment of desires? In this body, which is afflicted with desire, anger, greed, delusion, fear, despondency, envy, separation from the desirable, union with the undesirable, hunger, thirst, senility, death, disease, sorrow, and the like—what good is the enjoyment of desires?[5]

Life in the days when this was written was probably as close to nasty, brutish, and short as civilization ever was. There was no reason to hope to come back. So, how do we get out of these fetid shit bags? That brings us to the question of practices.

Practices

"The Self is indeed Brahman," the *Brihadaranyaka* tells us, "but through ignorance people identify it with intellect, mind, senses, passions, and the elements of earth, water, air, space, and fire."[6]

Okay. Now we know that we need to overcome our ignorance and learn to see the world and ourselves as they are, as the Sacred. But how do we do that? The Upanishads talk about a number of spiritual practices.

They recommend high moral standards, including right action, truthfulness, austerity, self-control, tranquility, and humaneness.[7] Other practices that are said to dispell our ignorance and guide us toward liberation include meditating on Om, being aware of our breathing, controlling the senses, discovering the different layers of the energy body, and labeling what we are *not* in order to know what we *are*. Ready?

Om

"Let us meditate on OM the imperishable, the beginning of prayer"; that is chapter one, verse one of the *Chandogya Upanishad.*[8]

Om is the most important mantra in yoga. In the Vedas, Om is used at the beginning and end of prayers and rituals to express awe and reverence, similar to the Christian use of amen. In the Upanishads, Om becomes much, much more.

Om is the sound of creation. When the sages turned deep within and listened to the infinite, they heard the sound Om. It is the *anahata*, the "unstruck" sound that pervades reality. It is also within each of us, deep within our hearts.

Om is the subject of the entire *Mandukya Upanishad,* where we learn that the sound of Om has four parts: A, U, M, and the silence that follows. These four parts correspond to the four states of consciousness: A to waking, U to dreaming, M to dreamless sleep, and silence to the state called simply *turiya,* the "fourth." Turiya is pure consciousness.

Om is everything. Om is Brahman and atman. Meditating on Om uses the sacred sound of creation to unlock the experience of ultimate reality.

Prana and Breath Awareness

The Upanishads also introduce the concept of prana. Prana is the life force of the universe. It is energy. Prana is the essence that animates all living beings. Every time we take a breath, we top up with prana, and prana is what leaves the body when we die.

Prana is attached to breath, and breath is attached to the mind. In the conversation between father and son, Uddalaka tells Shvetaketu,

> "It is like this. Take a bird that is tied with a string. It will fly off in every direction and, when it cannot find a resting-place anywhere else, it will alight back upon the very thing to which it is tied. Similarly, son, the mind flies off in every direction and, when it cannot find a resting-place anywhere else, it alights back upon the breath itself; for the mind, my son is tied to the breath."[9]

Because of this connection, it follows that if we can control the breath, then we can control our minds. This is the basis of pranayama.

Prana is both breath and energy. Brahman, as we saw earlier, is also energy. So prana, like all things, is Brahman. This leads to the statement in the *Kaushitaki Upanishad* that "Brahman is breath."[10] Not only does controlling the breath quiet the mind, but settle into the awareness of the flow of your breath and you will rest in Brahman. Our breath, the *Kaushitaki* says, is "the daily sacrifice offered internally."[11] Talking about inhalation and exhalation, it goes on, "One offers these two endless and deathless offerings without interruption, whether one is awake or asleep. All other offerings, on the other hand, are limited, for they consist of ritual activities."

In another half a millennium, pranayama will be one of the eight limbs of yoga in Patanjali's *Yoga Sutras*, and centuries after that it will be explored to its fullest in Hatha Yoga.

Controlling the Senses

Focusing on the sacred syllable Om and practicing breath awareness are both methods of turning inward, away from the constant stream of information bombarding our senses. In the Upanishads, this is the practice of yoga, variously interpreted by translators as concentration, meditation, and absorption.

The *Chandogya* explains why we want to gain control of our senses: "Control the senses and purify the mind. In a pure mind there is constant awareness of the Self. Where there is constant awareness of the Self, freedom ends bondage and joy ends sorrow."[12]

The practices of reciting Om and breath awareness help a seeker to control the senses and turn inward. It is then that spiritual development can begin in earnest.

Pancha Kosha

Pancha kosha (panca kosha) means "five sheaths" or "five casings." In English, they are often referred to as five bodies, probably because we think sheaths are for swords and casings are for sausages. The Upanishads' description of the pancha kosha is the first mention we have of the subtle body, also known as the energy body. The idea is that we each have these five bodies, nesting within each other, and each body is more subtle, energetically, than the previous.

Let's start with the text from the *Taittiriya Upanishad* where the sheaths are first mentioned:

> In the beginning this world was the non-
>   existent,
> And from it arose the existent.
> By itself it made a body for itself;
> Therefore it is called "well-made",

And precisely because it is well-made, it is the essence, for only when one has grasped that essence does one attain bliss. Now, who would breathe in, who would breathe out, if that essence were not there in space as bliss, for it is that essence that causes bliss. For when a man finds within that invisible, incorporeal, indistinct, and supportless essence, the fearless state on which to rest, then he becomes free from fear . . . .

After a man who knows this departs from this world—he first reaches the self (*ātman*) that consists of food, then the self that consists of lifebreath, then the self that consists of mind, then the self that consists of perception, and finally the self that consists of bliss. On this too we have the following verse:

> Before they reach it, words turn back,
> together with the mind;
> One who knows that bliss of *brahman*,
> he is never afraid.

He does not agonize, thinking: "Why didn't I do the right thing? Why did I do the wrong thing?" A man who knows this frees himself (*ātman*) from these two thoughts. From these two thoughts, indeed, a man who knows this frees himself. That is the hidden teaching (*upaniṣad*).[13]

While the text makes it pretty clear that we encounter these sheaths after dying an enlightened death, the pancha kosha have become an important part of the living practice of yoga. What follows are the layers from the outermost to the innermost. *Maya* means "appearance" and reminds us that each of these "bodies" is temporary and therefore only relatively real.

1. *Anna-maya-kosha*: Directly translated, this is the food-appearance-sheath. It is the material, physical body.
2. *Prana-maya-kosha* (prāna-maya-kosha): Prana, as we've seen, is the cosmic energy that sustains life; it occurs with the breath but is not identical to it. The prana body could be called the life energy body.
3. *Mano-maya-kosha*: Translated in the text above as "the self that consists of mind," this is where sensations and emotions are felt.
4. *Vijnana-maya-kosha* (vijñāna-maya-kosha): The wisdom body, this is where perception, understanding, and higher thinking occur.
5. *Ananda-maya-kosha* (ānanda-maya-kosha): The bliss body is the Self within all our other selves through which we participate in the dance of the Sacred.

In the progression of the spiritual quest, we become sensitive to each of these levels and how they can blossom, gradually moving inward toward the bliss of union.

The oldest known instance of the term "yoga" as a spiritual practice occurs here, in the *Taittiriya's* discussion of the pancha kosha:

> Within the mental sheath, made up of waves
> Of thought, there is contained the sheath of wisdom.
> It has the same form, with faith as the head,
> Righteousness as the right arm and truth as left.
> Practice of meditation [yoga] is its heart,
> And discrimination its foundation.[14]

Yoga is the heart of the wisdom body.

Neti, Neti

Now we have the tools to control our senses and a map of what we'll find when we turn inward. Next, we have to contend with what we find within.

In the *Brihadaranyaka Upanishad,* we hear the story of Yājñavalkya and Maitreyī. Yajnavalkya has reached the point in this life where he is ready to take sannyasa and devote himself solely to gaining moksha. He calls his two wives to him and says it's time to settle his property between them, just as if he had died.

Maitreyi states that she has no wish for his goods but instead would prefer to share his wisdom. Possessions will only make her wealthy, she knows, whereas spiritual knowledge will set her free. Yajnavalkya is delighted with Maitreyi's response and sets about teaching her what he knows about discovering the atman and gaining immortality, that is to say, eternal freedom from samsara in Brahman.

"You see, Maitreyī—it is one's self (ātman) which one should see and hear, and on which one should reflect and concentrate. For by seeing and hearing one's [atman], and by reflecting and concentrating on one's [atman], one gains the knowledge of this whole world..."

"About this self (ātman), one can only say 'not ---, not ---.' It is ungraspable, for it cannot be grasped. It is undecaying, for it is not subject to decay. Nothing sticks to it, for it does not stick to anything. It is not bound; yet it neither trembles in fear nor suffers injury.

"Look—by what means can one perceive the perceiver? There, I have given you the instructions, Maitreyī. That's all there is to immortality."[15]

"Not ---, not ---," is sometimes translated as "not this, not that," and in Sanskrit is "*neti, neti.*" "Neti, neti" is repeated three times in the *Brihadaranyaka*.

This is a remarkable early instance of the *via negativa*, which means describing something by saying what it is not, and in particular denying that a finite concept can define God or the Ultimate Reality.

"Neti, neti" is the basis of an important meditation

technique. In this practice one simply asks, "Who am I?" And because the atman cannot be described, to every answer that arises we can say, "not this, not that," eventually wearing through the ego personality to the radiant core of being.

Self-realization

Let's say we have followed all of this advice. We have controlled our senses by chanting Om and practicing awareness of our breath. We have turned within and navigated through the five bodies. And we have overcome the temporary, changeable ego personality.

Now what?

Now bliss!

What we are promised is the experience of union, yoga, the unitive state where our subjectivity merges into the all-pervasive sacred consciousness that is Brahman. In the *Brihadaranyaka* it is described like this:

As a man in the arms of his beloved is not aware of what is without and what is within, so a person in union with the Self is not aware of what is without and what is within, for in that unitive state all desires find their perfect fulfillment. There is no other desire that needs to be fulfilled, and one goes beyond sorrow.

In that unitive state there is neither father nor mother, neither worlds nor gods nor even scriptures. In that state there is neither thief nor slayer, neither low caste nor high, neither monk nor ascetic. The Self is beyond good and evil, beyond all the suffering of the human heart.

But where there is unity, one without a second, that is the world of Brahman. This is the supreme goal of life, the supreme treasure, the supreme joy. Those who do not seek this supreme goal live on but a fraction of this joy.

Those who realize the Self enter into the peace that brings complete self-control and perfect patience. They see themselves in everyone and everyone in themselves.[16]

From the Forest to the Battlefield

Thus is the hidden wisdom of the forest dwellers. Let go of your small self, your ego personality. It isn't real in any lasting way. It changes with time, with growth, with drugs and hard knocks to the head. What is real is that sacred energy-consciousness that we share in common with all of creation. Let go of the small self to get in touch with the higher Self, with Brahman.

But what about the rest of us? What about all of those people who, for whatever reason, are not off living in the forest, renouncing everything to pursue moksha? Are we stuck in samsara, collecting karma and sorrow? Our next chapter introduces yoga for the spiritual needs of people who choose to stay in the world. In terms of caste, the Upanishads were written by and for brahmins. The epics are all about warriors.

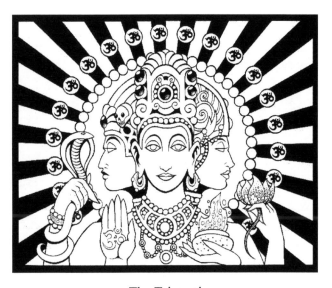

The Trimurti

3 GREAT WARRIORS
AND THE AGE OF EPICS

Next up in the history of yoga is the Epic Age, and is it ever! These sagas star brave, handsome men and strong, beautiful women who face avaricious humans and grotesque demons. They feature powerful gods, talking animals, and massive battles. And they always, always reward the good guy, eventually.

Trimurti

Before we get to the stories, we need to talk about the gods. While deities were central to the Vedas, the intentions behind the rituals were propitiation and supplication. In other words, rituals were meant to please the gods so they would give us what we need and take care of us. In the era of the epics, this relationship changes as Bhakti Yoga becomes a prominent spiritual path. In Bhakti Yoga, the yoga of divine love, the individual's or group's ishta devata is God with a capital "G" and is recognized as the Ultimate Power, worthy of complete devotion. Whereas in the Vedas the various gods are different faces of the One, in Bhakti Yoga, the devotee's chosen God *is* the One.

Vedic culture spread across the Indian subcontinent as tribes were conquered and brought under the domain of various kings. While there were beliefs that became marginalized, many local religious traditions merged with Vedic ideas and local gods merged with Vedic gods. One outcome of this coalescence has been called the ***trimurti***, the three forms, as seen in the illustration at the beginning of this chapter. The trimurti isn't so much worshipped as such; it's more a convenient categorization tool for the gods who became the three main deities of Hinduism: Brahma, Vishnu, and Shiva. They are the creator, the maintainer, and the destroyer, respectively. (The god Brahma is different from Brahman, the ultimate sacred substance of all that is, and both are separate from the priests who are called brahmins.) Each of the trimurti has distinguishing characteristics.

Brahma is the creator. He is pictured with four faces, looking in each of the four directions. He carries a container of water, out of which creation emanates. His consort is the goddess Sarasvati, the great river deified. She is the goddess of knowledge, music, and the arts. All gods have vehicles, and Brahma's is a swan.

Vishnu is the maintainer or preserver of creation. He is the god of dharma. To act according to one's dharma in the worldview of the epics means everything from respecting custom in social conduct, to following the livelihood and traditions of your caste, to righteousness and virtue. Vishnu is blue skinned, as are all of his earthly incarnations, a.k.a. **avatars**. His consort is Lakshmi, goddess of beauty and fortune, and his vehicle is Garuda, a large bird-like creature. (Garudasana or eagle pose is named after him.)

And Shiva is the destroyer. He wears a snake around his neck, a symbol of alert stillness and general badassery. Shiva is the Lord of Animals and the Lord of Yoga. His skin is gray with the ashes of the dead, a constant reminder of the impermanence of life. His consort is Parvati, goddess of love, fertility, and devotion. They have two sons, Ganesha and Kartikeya. The elephant-headed Ganesha is the remover of obstacles and god of intellect and wisdom, and Kartikeya, who also goes by Marugan, Skandan, Kumaran, and quite a few other names, is the god of war. Shiva's vehicle is the bull, Nandi.

Each of these deities has libraries of mythology about them that are fascinating, with much of it gathered in the extensive *Puranas*. While the underlying truth that there is one God with many faces remains, various denominations hold that their chosen God, for the most part either Vishnu or Shiva, is that one God, and other gods are other faces their God takes on.

In this chapter we will be introduced to two incarnations of Vishnu: Rama and Krishna. Those are the avatars whose deeds are recorded in the two great epics of India, the *Ramayana* and the *Mahabharata*. First we'll look at the Rama saga; then a brief look at the storyline of the *Mahabharata*; and finally we'll dive into the *Bhagavad Gita*, a book within the *Mahabharata* and one of the most important texts in the yoga tradition.

The Ramayana

One of the oldest epics on earth, the *Ramayana* is still being read, recited, chanted, sung, danced, enacted on stage and in shadow puppet theaters, filmed for television and Bollywood movies, made into graphic novels, and used as a theme for video games. It is loved.

Beginning

The story starts like this: Rama is the son of Dasharatha, king of Ayodhya. Rama is beloved by all for his gentle and compassionate nature and his respect for dharma. He is married to the beautiful Sita, who was found as a child and raised by King Janaka, the ruler of a neighboring province.

On the eve of Rama's coronation as crown prince, King Dasharatha's youngest and favorite wife, under the influence of her evil servant, becomes jealous and demands that Dasharatha grant her the two boons he had promised when she saved his life several years previously. She insists that Rama be sent to the forest for fourteen years and her own son be named crown prince.

Dasharatha is devastated, but Rama agrees to go willingly to protect his father's dharma. Perhaps you are picking up that dharma is a theme here.

The *Ramayana* is seven books long. So far, I've summarized the first two books, the *Book of Childhood* and the *Book of Ayodhya*. There are many other characters, including Rama's brothers, Sita's family, and the other queens. There are servants, ministers of state, and sages, including the *kulaguru*, or clan's spiritual teacher, Vasishtha (Vāsiṣṭha).

Think *Game of Thrones*–style epic, with complex interweaving storylines chock full of good and evil, joy and sorrow, violence and gore, magic and supernatural feats, sexual tension, demons who drink blood and eat humans, and good guys who, well, just check out this passage where Rama is proving his skill to Sugriva, king of the monkey people, who are called *vanaras*:

> He [Rama] strung his bow so quickly the vanaras stepped back a pace from him. Rama bent his bow in a circle and shot one arrow of uncanny trajectory through all seven trees. Sugriva gave a hoarse cry. His monkeys leaped into the air, gibbering in amazement. Rama's arrow, which had entered the earth beyond the seventh sala [tree], flew up from the ground behind him and settled back into his quiver.[1]

Yeah, he's that kind of hero.

Middle

The third book, the *Book of the Forest*, describes the years Rama, Sita, and Rama's brother Lakshmana spend in exile. The men dress as forest-dwelling ascetics, with their dreadlocks piled on top of their heads. They lead an idyllic existence and defeat evil when it crosses their path.

One of these evils is the bloodthirsty demon, or *rak-shasi,* Surpanakha. Surpanakha is the sister of Ravana, king of all *rakshasas* and of Lanka (modern-day Sri Lanka). In the long-distant past, Ravana performed extreme austerities and won a boon from Brahma, the creator god; now Ravana cannot be defeated in battle by any god or other supernatural being. He has been terror-izing creation for thousands of years.

Surpanakha is smitten with Rama and Lakshmana. She takes on a beautiful form and offers herself as a wife first to Rama and, when he teases and rebuffs her, then to Lakshmana. Because she is forward and crude, the brothers recognize her as a *rakshasi* and Lakshamana hacks off her ears and her nose. Thus mutilated, Surpan-akha flees back to her clan with whom she lives in the forest and provokes a war between the rakshasas and Rama. Rama defeats this rakshasa army, thousands of demons, single-handedly.

Surpanakha takes news of these events to her brother. She wants Ravana to exact revenge for her, but Ravana only becomes interested when he hears of Sita's beauty. He decides he must have her for his harem. At the end of book three, Sita is kidnapped by the demon king.

The fourth book is the *Book of Kishkinda,* the mon-key kingdom. It describes the search for Sita, in which Rama and Lakshmana join forces with the vanaras, an ape-like race often described as monkey people, and some well-spoken bears. Book five, the *Book of Beauty,* is all about Hanuman, one of the vanaras. It is Hanuman who finds Sita on Lanka.

Book six is the *Book of War*, in which there is a truly epic series of battles between Ravana's rakshasas and Rama and the vanaras. There is carnage and death, illusion and healing, until finally (spoiler!) Ravana is defeated.

End

Patriarchy AF

Upon being reunited with Sita, Rama spurns her, asking how it could possibly be dharma for him to take back a wife who has lived in another man's palace. To prove her purity, Sita steps into a raging fire and walks out unharmed. The whole party returns to Ayodhya, and there is much rejoicing.

Book seven is sometimes called the *Book of the North* and sometimes simply the *Last Book*. In it we see Rama installed as king. He discovers that some of his subjects question Sita's chastity and sends her away, pregnant as she is. In some iterations, Rama asks Lakshmana to kill her. In these versions, Lakshmana does not kill Sita but brings Rama the heart of a deer or the blood of a rabbit instead.

Sita gives birth to twins who eventually grow to (a) take revenge on their father for discarding their mother or (b) participate in a happy family reunion and (c) sometimes both.

So ends the story of Rama.

Which *Ramayana*?

As we can tell from the multiple endings, there are several variations of the story. While the historical families on which the Rama saga is based probably lived around 2500 BCE, the oldest written version of the story dates to around the 4th century BCE and is attributed to Valmiki. Written in Sanskrit and in verse form, *Valmiki's Ramayana* claims the full seven books. Though textual analysis shows that the first and seventh books were added later, tradition holds that the entire poem was written by one person.

In *Valmiki's Ramayana*, Rama is recognized as an incarnation of Vishnu. Vishnu, in his role as the maintainer, comes to earth as an avatar when humankind needs help maintaining order or dharma. In this case, he takes human form so that Ravana can be defeated. However, throughout the story, Rama doesn't seem to remember he's an avatar. Instead he is held forth as the ideal man who puts dharma first and foremost in every aspect of his life.

Another Sanskrit version is the much shorter *Adhyatma Ramayana*, or *Spiritual Ramayana*, which is part of the *Brahmanda Purana* and was probably written during the 1st century CE. In this one, Rama is overtly and repeatedly praised as Vishnu's avatar from the moment of his birth. This iteration likely reveals the transition from Vishnu being a minor deity at the end of the Vedic era, when *Valmiki's Ramayana* was set down, to Vishnu as the supreme God for many throughout the Indian subcontinent some four hundred years later.

Through the millennia, the story and the stories within the story moved throughout the populace of Southern Asia orally, leading to regional variations. In the 12th century CE, the scholar and poet Kandam wrote a Tamil language version, the *Ramavatharam*, which is still popular among Tamil speakers today. In the 16th century, the poet-saint Tulsidas wrote *Ramcharitmanas*, which means "Lake of the Deeds of Rama," in a vernacular form of Hindi. This is the version from which most television and movie Ramayanas draw.

Today there are variations of the Rama saga based on region, language, age, gender, social status, politics, medium, and even religion, as there are Buddhist and Jain versions as well as Muslim interpretations, too. It would be hard to overstate the role of *The Ramayana* in South Asia.

Why Read It?

There are times when the *Ramayana* glaringly highlights how morals change over time. In Valmiki's version, Sita is more outspoken; in Tulsidas' she is more demure, reflecting the cultural ideals about virtuous women of each era. Throughout the books, a present-day reader is likely to trip over virtues surrounding sex and gender that remind us that this story comes from a strikingly different time. But is still wrong.

Even in the context of its land of origin, there are episodes that centuries of revisionists have struggled to reframe to put Rama in a better light. One instance of this is when he kills the king of the monkeys from hiding instead of facing him in battle. Another is when he angrily rebukes Sita even though he supposedly knows she was entirely faithful. But what's more amazing than the differences between what was heroic then and what is heroic now is how often the dharma Rama seeks to uphold matches up with our current standards of right action and cosmic justice.

There are a number of reasons to read the *Ramayana*: it's a great story; it's entertaining and an ancient masterwork; it's a window to the past and to the present as it is culturally relevant to hundreds of millions, possibly billions, of people; and finally, it makes us question our own dharma. What does it mean to be virtuous? What was I brought here to do? What role do I play in this universal dance?

The Yoga of the Ramayana

Whenever I read an ancient yogic text, I'm on the alert for signs of anything similar to what is passed on as yoga in America these days. Through modern postural yoga we are familiar with the names of Hanuman (through hanumanasana a.k.a. the splits) and Vasishtha (through vasishthasana a.k.a. side plank). And these postures take on new meaning when you know the stories behind them. Also of interest is that the Ramayana contains the first references we've come across to **surya namaskara** (sūrya nāmaskara) or sun salutations. While there are no descriptions of the ritual actions involved, Rama and Lakshmana perform surya namaskara more than once and always while standing waist deep in water. So, obviously, not the same surya namaskara that we're doing at the flow class down at the local studio.

As for where it stands on the philosophy of yoga, Rama follows the wisdom of the Upanishads, and pieces of its philosophy are sprinkled throughout. We are reminded that change is the only constant and death the only certainty in this life, and that we all reap the fruit of our karma. While in the forest, Rama, Sita, and Lakshmana meet wise sages and groups of sannyasins whom they protect and from whom they learn.

But Rama is not a renunciate, he just lives like one for a very long time. Through it all, he never ceases to be a warrior or a married man. He is *passionate*. At one point Rama reminds the leader of the vanaras, "My friend, dharma [duty], artha [wealth, power], and kama [pleasure] should be of equal importance in one's life." Rama is an example of how to *live*, not how to escape the wheel of samsara.

The Shudra

Toward the end of the *Ramayana* there is an interesting vignette concerning a renunciate of the shudra caste. Shudras were the lowest varna, the servant class, and were not supposed to perform tapas. Spiritual liberation came after being reincarnated as one of the higher castes, and to act above your caste was a sin.

Rama, who is now the king, is told that because of this great sin being performed in his land a brahmin's son has died. He finds the sannyasin, as we read in Ramesh Menon's contemporary version, "standing upon his head in sirsasana below that tree, in intense tapasya."

Rama asks why he practices such a severe austerity and what caste he is from. "I am a shudra, Rama; my name is Sambuka," comes the sannyasin's even reply. "And I stand up on my head in dhyana [meditation] because I want to conquer Devaloka [the land of the gods] and be Lord of the four quarters."

Rama decapitates him. The gods of Devaloka, including Indra and Agni, appear and praise Rama for upholding the dharma. The brahmin's son returns to life.

"But as he wiped his blade clean on some long grass, Rama had tears in his eyes."[2]

The *Ramayana* is about following one's dharma, whether you like it or not. As we will see, the *Bhagavad Gita* is about that, too. But the *Gita* adds the depth of Karma Yoga to the practice. Not only should we do our duty and maintain righteousness in the world, but we should do so with no expectations.

The Mahabharata

The second epic is the *Mahabharata,* which is an enormous eighteen books long. The name comes from *maha,* which means "great," and Bharata, which was the name of the king who founded the dynasty the book follows. The central story has been dated back to 1500 BCE, but along the way, it *collected.* Just like the religious traditions of Hinduism, the *Mahabharata* gathered together what people found useful and important enough to warrant remembering, in this case traditional tales and morality plays. This went on as the story spread throughout the subcontinent until the

Mahabharata reached its current gigantic form around 400 CE.

At its heart, it is a story about the descendants of a man named Vyasa, who plays two important roles. The name Vyasa means "compiler," and he is credited with dictating the *Mahabharata* to Ganesha. The story goes they made a deal: Vyasa would tell the whole saga in one sitting so long as Ganesha would only write it down with full understanding of each word. Ganesha's quill broke part way through the transcription, so he snapped off one of his tusks and continued by using it as his writing utensil.

Besides being the author of the *Mahabharata*, Vyasa is also a character within it. In the story, he is a king who has two sons. The older brother, who would have rightfully become king, abdicates because he is blind, so the younger brother becomes king instead. Both brothers have sons, and they all live peacefully at court. The cousins grow up together, sharing all of their experiences. They have the same teachers and weapons trainers, and together they learn what it means to be kshatriya, of the warrior caste.

Then, the sons of the older brother become greedy, and the story becomes one of good versus evil, right versus wrong.

The core of the *Mahabharata* is the story of these two groups of cousins: the treachery of the older brother's sons, called the Kauravas, and the valor of the younger brother's sons, the Pandavas. The Kauravas cheat the Pandavas out of their lands and dishonor them by shaming their wife, Draupadi, at a public gathering.

The Pandavas have to live in exile as forest dwellers for twelve years and in hiding for another year after that.

When they return, the Kauravas renege on their agreement to give the Pandavas back their land and the cousins go to war.

Krishna the Charioteer

As the two sides are gearing up for battle, both seek the support of Krishna, who is king of the nearby territory of Dwaraka. Arjuna, the great archer from the Pandava family, and Duryodhana, the eldest Kaurava brother, seek him out simultaneously. Krishna agrees to help them both. To one, he says, he will give his army of a million men. The other he will accompany, but he will not fight in the war. He will simply be on the side of the one who chooses him.

Arjuna gets first choice and chooses Krishna without any hesitation. And that is how Krishna, avatar of Vishnu, comes to be Arjuna's charioteer.

While the armies are lining up on the battlefield, Arjuna asks Krishna to take him to the middle of the field so he can see who he will be fighting. When they get there, Arjuna looks into the faces of his family members, friends, and teachers, and he loses the will to fight. How, he asks, can it be right to kill people he loves? He would rather die himself, he says, than kill them. He lets his bow slide from his hand and he weeps.

Krishna gently reminds Arjuna of what he already knows, that the soul cannot die. What he kills on the battlefield, what plays out in this human drama, has no bearing on the eternal substance of the people involved. They are manifesting their karma on this plane and will come back and do it again. And while Arjuna may yearn to renounce this life, he cannot escape his dharma. But he can practice yoga, which Krishna defines as "perfect evenness of mind." Renunciation is not only for the sannyasin. One can practice yoga while performing one's dharma by renouncing, or becoming detached, from the outcome of one's actions. ↗in Mahabharta

This is how the *Bhagavad Gita* or *Song of the Lord* begins. The rest is a record of the conversation through which Krishna guides Arjuna to understand the real battle, the spiritual struggle within.

If the Bhagavad Gita Were a Color

The *Gita*, as it is affectionately called, is one of the most beloved spiritual texts ever. There are a number of reasons why it resonates with so many people on such a deep level. First, whereas the Vedas were the property of the elite priestly caste, and the Upanishads were reserved for forest dwelling sannyasins, the *Gita* speaks to people who choose to play their roles in society while still following a spiritual path. Secondly, as we will see, it gives options. There isn't just one way to earn salvation. Just as we have different personalities and inclinations, we need different paths and practices to guide us to the Sacred. Thirdly, it is unambiguous—it leaves no room for hesitation about good versus evil or about right action.

Trying to summarize the *Bhagavad Gita* is like trying to describe a new color or taste—doomed to fall far short of the actual experience. It is something you must read for yourself. All I can hope to do here is introduce the new ideas and look at how they fit in with what has come before. First we'll look at the main philosophical concepts and worldview of the *Gita*. Then we'll see how it brings together Jnana, Karma, and Bhakti Yogas. Finally, we'll learn what wisdom and liberation look like from a bhakti perspective.

The "G" Word

The philosophy of the *Gita* begins and ends with God. For some seekers, this is a turn off. Many people who are drawn to American yoga came to Eastern philosophies because of a need that was unfulfilled by Western religion, especially Christianity. We've been told a lot of things about God, and for some the word itself causes a certain amount of distress. As we will see later, when Hinduism and yoga first came to America, Bhakti Yoga was roundly ignored. It's as if we'd had enough of a (distorted) personal relationship with the Divine and needed something more abstract and less emotional. If that's where you are, you're not alone.

In the *Bhagavad Gita*, God is Brahman, the eternal, changeless Reality. God is the Supreme Spirit, the immortal, transcendent Self. God created the universe and pervades it. God both fills the universe and vastly exceeds it. And God is within each of us. So, if you are struggling with the God concept, it can help to simply replace that word with the one that works for you: maybe Brahman, the Sacred, the Really Real, Consciousness, Energy, or Love.

The Gunas

To continue with the philosophy of the *Gita*, God is what *is*, but we are ignorant of this because we are blinded by the **gunas** or qualities of nature. Everything in the cosmos, in nature, is created by the interplay of these three primary forces—everything, including the mind. Here again we run into what I think is one of the most interesting differences between Hindu and Western metaphysics. As mentioned in chapter 2, in Western philosophy, from the Age of Reason on, we've put mind and matter into separate categories. That's the Western dualism: body vs. spirit; matter vs. mind. In yoga at this point, the two categories are *Purusha* and **prakriti**. We have seen this word "Purusha" in the chapter on the Vedas, where it referred to the Cosmic Man. Over time, especially through the Upanishads, the meaning attached to Purusha evolved. Now it is all-encompassing. Purusha has become another name for the Sacred, the Absolute. Prakriti means creation, and creation includes both mind and matter.

As we have begun to see, in most branches of yoga philosophy, any separation between Purusha and prakriti, the Sacred and creation, is overcome by the recognition that creation emanates from and is part of the Sacred. There are not two substances; there is only the Sacred. In the later terminology of Vedanta, the Sacred is **satchitananda** (satcitānanda), "being-consciousness-bliss"; it is the energy of which all things are made. And once we identify energy as consciousness, and remember that matter is simply energy at a slower vibratory rate, the ontological difference between matter and mind disappears. We'll return to this idea in later chapters. Right now, back to the gunas.

The three gunas are *sattva*, *rajas*, and *tamas*.

Sattva is the principle of lucidity. It refers to all that is pure, bright, and illuminating. Someone who is sattvic is what we might consider spiritual or saintly.

Rajas is the principle of dynamism. Rajas is all about motion, energy, and activation. A person dominated by rajas might be easily excited, anxious, or passionate.

Tamas is the principle of inertia. Think slowness, decay, and restriction. A person dominated by tamas would exhibit sloth and resistance.

Because of these three forces, we experience the emotional drives of attachments and aversions. Tamas makes us not want to get out of bed, take risks, etc.; rajas makes us strive for connection, recognition, etc.; and sattva makes us seek spiritual growth and experience inner peace. In fact, everything we think we are is really just the play of the gunas, as Krishna tells Arjuna:

All actions are performed by the gunas of prakriti. Deluded by identification with the ego, a person thinks, "*I* am the doer." But the illumined man or woman understands the domain of the gunas and is not attached. Such people know that the gunas interact with each other; they do not claim to be the doer.[3]

Jnana Yoga

Through the actions of the gunas, the sacred reality is hidden from us behind the created world of mind and matter. Because the gunas color everything we see, we give this changeable, temporary, surface world far more importance than it's due. And this attribution of significance leads to sorrow. What we are attached to always deserts us eventually. What we are averse to, we must suffer through. As long as we are under the sway of the gunas, we continue to create karma and stay on the wheel of rebirth.

Hopefully this is starting to sound familiar. It's the same idea as in the Upanishads—because of our ignorance we are stuck in samsara. And, also like in the Upanishads, the *Gita* tells us that to dispel our ignorance and avoid sorrow and suffering, we should seek to see past the material world and into the truth about God. Further still, the *Gita* also advises us to control our senses and develop one-pointed concentration, in other words, to practice meditation.

Krishna advocates these practices of Jnana Yoga when he tells Arjuna:

The practice of meditation frees one from all affliction. This is the path of yoga. Follow it with determination and sustained enthusiasm. Renouncing wholeheartedly all selfish desires and expectations, use your will to control the senses. Little by little, through patience and repeated effort, the mind will become stilled in the Self.[4]

One significant difference between the Upanishads and the *Gita* is that here we are encouraged to give up "all selfish desires" rather than our place in the world. This fits in with its broader message about Karma Yoga.

Karma Yoga

Karma Yoga is an all-encompassing approach to walking the spiritual path while maintaining our worldly roles. Sometimes, these days, we see Karma Yoga used in the sense of volunteerism or selfless service. Really, a better word for that would be *seva*.

The foundation of Karma Yoga is virtuous action. It's important to recognize that mental and verbal actions count too. That is to say, Karma Yoga applies to thought, speech, and deed.

So, what does it mean to act virtuously? In addition to "renouncing wholeheartedly selfish desires," Krishna gives Arjuna this list of virtues to maintain and qualities to avoid:

Be fearless and pure; never waver in your determination or your dedication to the spiritual life. Give freely. Be self-controlled, sincere, truthful, loving, and full of the desire to serve. Realize the truth of the scriptures; learn to be detached and take joy in renunciation. Do not get angry or harm any living creature, but be compassionate and gentle; show good will to all. Cultivate vigor, patience, will, purity; avoid malice and pride. Then, Arjuna, you will achieve your divine destiny. Other qualities, Arjuna, make a person more and more inhuman: hypocrisy, arrogance, conceit, anger, cruelty, ignorance.[5]

A little later Krishna goes on about qualities to avoid:

There are three gates to this self-destructive hell: lust, anger, and greed. Renounce these three. Those who escape from these three gates of darkness, Arjuna, seek what is best and attain life's supreme goal.[6]

Loka samgraha is another virtue that is called out. It translates as "world gathering" and embodies the concept that actions ought to promote the welfare of all beings and the good of the whole world. "The ignorant work for their own profit, Arjuna," Krishna tells him, "the wise work for the welfare of the world, without thought for themselves."[7] And the benefit of loka samgraha is illustrated when Krishna says, "Strive constantly to serve the welfare of the world; by devotion to selfless work one attains the supreme goal of life."[8]

Loka samgraha and admonitions to be compassionate toward all beings are balanced by an equal emphasis on remaining detached, which goes hand in hand with renouncing the outcome or fruits of one's actions.

> Seek refuge in the attitude of detachment and you will amass the wealth of spiritual awareness. Those who are motivated only by desire for the fruits of action are miserable, for they are constantly anxious about the results of what they do. When consciousness is unified, however, all vain anxiety is left behind. There is no cause for worry, whether things go well or ill. Therefore, devote yourself to the discipline of yoga, for yoga is skill in action.[9]

Dharma

Also necessary to Karma Yoga and living a virtuous life is maintaining your own dharma. As we've seen, "dharma" means "duty," but what is duty? To do what is expected of us, what culture says is correct, or what we feel or know intuitively to be right? And how do we know what our individual dharma might be?

In the epics, dharma refers to duty on several planes. First, it means upholding personal morality; next, respecting social traditions; and ultimately, maintaining rita or cosmic order.

Our dharma plays out through our life circumstances, both internally, in the way the gunas manifest as our personalities, and externally, in our cultural and environmental conditions. These circumstances are what they are due to our karma. Shirking our dharma squanders this opportunity to work through and "burn up" the seeds of karma that keep us tethered to samsara.

And while the situation of our current manifestation may seem less than ideal or maybe even a bad fit, according to the *Gita* it is better to work within our current circumstances than to waste this chance by wishing or even pretending it were otherwise:

> It is better to perform one's own duties imperfectly than to master the duties of another. By fulfilling the obligations he is born with, a person never comes to grief. No one should abandon duties because he sees defects in them. Every action, every activity, is surrounded by defects as a fire is surrounded by smoke.[10]

The grass may be greener on the other side of the fence, but it's not your grass.

Bhakti Yoga

Besides the right knowledge and meditation of Jnana Yoga and Karma Yoga's virtuous, detached action, Krishna also offers the devotion of Bhakti Yoga as an option for dispelling our ignorance, seeing through the gunas, and gaining spiritual liberation.

Bhakti Yoga includes all of the God-oriented rituals, prayers, and mantras. Krishna tells Arjuna to keep God always in mind, and that this is the best and most accessible path:

> Whatever you do, make it an offering to me—the food you eat, the sacrifices you make, the help you

give, even your suffering. In this way you will be freed from the bondage of karma, and from its results both pleasant and painful. Then, firm in renunciation and yoga, with your heart free, you will come to me.[11]

Emphasizing the omnipotence and oneness of God, Krishna tells Arjuna that even those who worship other gods are worshipping him because there is only one God. It isn't important which path a person picks, Krishna says, as long as they are doing spiritual work. "As they approach me, so I receive them. All paths, Arjuna, lead to me."[12]

These different paths—Jnana, Karma, and Bhakti—are not exclusive of one another. While different personalities will be called more in one direction than another, it is common to practice a mixture of two or even all three. And the result of all spiritual practice, according to the *Gita*, is wisdom.

Traits of the Wise

Throughout the conversation, Arjuna repeatedly asks Krishna how we can tell if someone is making progress on the path. What does a holy person look like? How do they act? Krishna tells him a wise person is free from fear, has peace of mind, and understands that all beings are part of the one interconnected whole:

The infinite joy of touching Brahman is easily attained by those who are free from the burden of evil and established within themselves. They see the Self in every creature and all creation in the Self. With consciousness unified through meditation, they see everything with an equal eye.[13]

Above all, the enlightened person possesses equanimity:

When you are unmoved by the confusion of ideas and your mind is completely united in deep samadhi [unitive consciousness]; you will attain the state of perfect yoga . . . . [W]hen you move amidst the world of sense, free from attachment and aversion alike, there comes the peace in which all sorrows end, and you live in the wisdom of the Self.[14]

And one last example that summarizes the qualities of wisdom:

Healed of their sins and conflicts, working for the good of all beings, the holy sages attain nirvana in Brahman. Free from anger and selfish desire, unified in mind, those who follow the path of yoga and realize the Self are established forever in that supreme state.[15]

Release from Samsara

As we enter the discussion of liberation in the *Gita*, we find another issue, like renunciation, where there are differences of opinion according to various yogic paths. And that issue is this: can liberation occur while we are living, or do we have to die that one final death in order to be free from the cycle of rebirth? According to the *Gita*, the wise person who maintains one-pointed concentration on God as they die will merge with God and escape samsara.

> This supreme Lord who pervades all existence, the true Self of all creatures, may be realized through undivided love. There are two paths, Arjuna, which the soul may follow at the time of death. One leads to rebirth and the other to liberation.[16]

Or said this way:

> The Lord is the supreme poet, the first cause, the sovereign ruler, subtler than the tiniest particle, the support of all, inconceivable, bright as the sun beyond darkness. Remembering him in this way at the time of death, through devotion and the power of meditation, with your mind completely stilled and your concentration fixed in the center of spiritual awareness between the eyebrows, you will realize the supreme Lord.[17]

Later traditions will hold that living beings can be enlightened, but for the *Gita*, as well as for the upcoming *Yoga Sutras*, to escape the cycle of birth, life, death, and rebirth, this life has to end.

Americans and the *Gita*

In my experience, I've found that some American yogis, when reading the *Gita* for the first time, are left with a bad taste in their mouth. Especially depending on the translation, the *Gita* can come across as didactic and authoritarian. In other words, a lot like the repressive forms of religion many of us seek to outgrow. And here we thought yoga was about spirituality and personal growth, when it turns out it's all about war and dharma and maintaining the social order? Sheez. If that's what I was looking for, I'd be a fundamentalist!

And yes, the *Gita* can be interpreted that way. But it can also be taken as saying the roles we play in life are secondary to our true nature. Whatever crap we have to put up with, through yoga we can be inwardly established in peace and joy. And that is really what all yoga is about.

Epic Yoga

In the Upanishads, yoga referred to the practices of sense control, concentration, and absorption, in another word, meditation. By the time of the epics, its meaning was vastly expanded. The word "yoga" appears dozens of times in the *Bhagavad Gita.* It is defined as "perfect evenness of mind" and "skill in action." It refers to various paths of spiritual pursuit, the act of meditation, and the equanimity we can achieve through spiritual practice. Yoga is the path, the practice, and the state of consciousness associated with liberation.

As we move forward through the timeline, into the *Yoga Sutras* of Patanjali (Patañjali), these new definitions of yoga come with us.

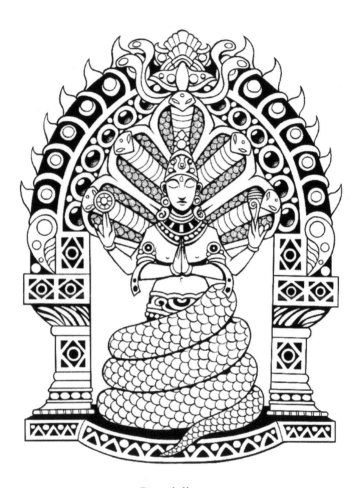

Patanjali

4 KRIYA AND ASHTANGA YOGA IN PATANJALI'S *YOGA SUTRAS*

If you've been around the yoga-sphere for more than a couple of seconds, you've probably heard of Patanjali's *Yoga Sutras,* a.k.a. Classical Yoga. The *Sutras* are the go-to philosophical guide for most schools of American yoga. In our chronology, the *Sutras* mark the transition from BCE to probably around the second century this side of Jesus.

According to the mythology that grew up around him, Patanjali was an incarnation of Ananta Shesha, the serpent who serves as Vishnu's couch between world cycles. In the story, a yogini named Goniki prays for a son to whom she can pass along her wisdom. As she prays, she holds her hands with her palms together in *anjali* mudra. Anjali means "offering," and the mudra is a symbol of reverence and honoring. When she opens her hands, there is a tiny snake who then becomes a human child. Ananta Shesha has fallen to earth. The

Sanskrit word for fallen is *pat*, so the name can be seen to mean fallen (pat) offering (anjali). Patanjali is often depicted with the lower half of a snake, hinting at his true form as Ananta Shesha.

We know very little about the historical Patanjali. We can safely assume he was a sage and a teacher. And we know he didn't develop the ideas he wrote about so much as compile the key elements of yoga theory and practice as they were conceived in his day. The text contains 195 or 196 (depending on the source) aphorisms or **sutras**. The word *sutra* comes from the same root as the English word "suture." It means thread. Each thread or aphorism is meant to be a learning tool, to be given due consideration, unwoven and pondered—the opposite of an overview, which is what we're doing here!

Within the *Sutras,* Patanjali talks about two different schools of yoga: **Kriya** and **Ashtanga**. Kriya means action specifically devoted to spiritual development and ashtanga means eight limbs. We'll cover both—first Kriya, then Ashtanga.

Early commentaries on this text are lost. There are hundreds of years between the *Sutras* and the first extant writings explaining and ruminating on its meaning. So, what those of Patanjali's time would have learned from their guru as they worked through the text is largely a matter of speculation. We are, however, already familiar with the fundamentals of the worldview within which Patanjali wrote: life is full of suffering because we mistake what is temporary and created for what is ultimate and enduring. Patanjali uses the terminology

Purusha and prakriti, with Purusha referring to the Self or transcendental consciousness and prakriti to the created cosmos or nature, which includes both matter and mind.

We saw in the Upanishads how our ignorance of the Sacred leads to attachments and aversions, to karma, and to continued incarnations in samsara. Patanjali adds that it also leads to deepening our *samskara*, which are psychological imprints or habits of mind. These deeply rooted tendencies of thought may come from previous lives or from this one. To overcome our ignorance and our samskara, we must engage in ***abhyasa*** (abhyāsa) or spiritual practice, and cultivate an attitude of ***vairagya*** (vairāgya), which is detachment or dispassion.

What follows is my best effort to summarize the main ideas and the philosophical feel of the *Sutras*. There are roughly 108 billion English translations of the *Sutras*, give or take. I've relied on three, those of Georg Feuerstein, Chip Hartranft, and Rama Prasad. The *Yoga Sutras* are separated into four chapters or ***padas***, which means "feet." We will travel though each one in turn.

Samadhi Pada

The first chapter goes right for the gold and tells us the goal of Kriya Yoga is to calm the mind in order to undo our samskara and become a mirror for the sacred reality, Purusha. I'm not going to go line by line, but let's do look at the first two sentences.

95

The first line of the *Sutras* says, "Now, the teachings of yoga." That was the traditional way to start a work like this.

The second sentence, *yogas citta vrtti nirodhah*, has been variously translated.

~ "Yoga is the restriction (nirodha) of the fluctuations of consciousness (citta)," Feuerstein[1]
~ "Yoga is to still the patterning of consciousness," Hartranft[2]
~ "Yoga is the restraint of mental modifications," Prasad[3]

In other words, the goal of yoga is to still the mind. We usually think we are the mind. But, as we've seen, we can't be the mind because the mind isn't anything enduring. It's all perception, interpretation, and memory. None of it is lasting. Mindstuff is as fickle and ephemeral as anything else in the created world of prakriti.

Patanjali tells us that when yoga works and the mind is still, that's when we discover samadhi. Samadhi is the state of unified consciousness, sometimes translated as integration or ecstasy. It is not a permanent state. It is a place we can visit that helps move us toward freedom from samsara.

Lists

The samadhi pada is big on lists. The first one we come across is the list of the five types of mental activity. They are right perception, misperception, imagination, deep sleep, and memory. According to Patanjali, to overcome these mental states and reach samadhi we must practice (list number two) devotion, reciting Om, and meditation. Okay, but devotion to whom? Patanjali uses the word ***Ishvara*** (Īshvara), which means Lord. Through a close reading we find that he meant it as a special instance of Purusha or Self that is utterly separate from the created world. This is super abstract, and many practicing yogis today prefer the concept of ishta devata, or worshipping the divine in the form of one's chosen deity.

So, we are to practice devotion, recite Om, and meditate in order to still the mind. But there are distractions, which he also lists (in list number three): sickness, apathy, doubt, carelessness, laziness, sexual indulgence, delusion, lack of progress along the path, and the inability to maintain progress when we achieve it. Along with these distractions, there are the physical symptoms of being distracted (list number four): pain, depression, shakiness, and unsteady breathing.

Patanjali then lists four practices to overcome the distractions (list number five):

1. cultivate friendliness, compassion, gladness, and equanimity toward all things
2. practice pranayama
3. reflect on the insights from dreams
4. practice meditation

After all these lists—the five types of mental activity, the three practices to overcome them, the nine mental and four physical distractions, and the four practices to overcome the distractions—we end up back again at meditation. It is the central practice of Kriya Yoga and deserves close attention. It is here in the *Sutras* that we learn about ***samyama***, the process of meditation.

Samyama

There are three stages or parts of the process of sam-yama and they flow together fluidly. They are ***dharana***, *dhyana*, and samadhi.

First, in dharana or concentration, we sit down to meditate by focusing the mind on something, maybe the breath, a mantra, or the example I'll use here, a candle flame. There will be distractions, especially in the form of thoughts: thoughts about other people, stuff we need to do, pets interrupting us, maybe even thoughts about the fact that we're meditating, wondering how it's going and if we're doing it right. If we stick with it, we let these thoughts go and keep coming back to the object of meditation, the candle flame. Dharana is the only step we have control over. The next two either happen or they don't. All we can do is set the stage.

The second step is dhyana, which is often translated as meditation or absorption. Here, we become completely absorbed in the object of meditation. The distractions are gone, and meditation is effortless. In this state, only the subject (you) and the object (candle flame) are present in consciousness.

Finally, in the unitive consciousness of samadhi, there is no distinction between subject and object. The ego personality is completely transcended; there is only ecstasy and bliss.

Patanjali describes two types of samadhi: *samprajnata* (samprajnāta) and *asamprajnata* (asamprajnāta), which can be thought of as with and without cognition, respectively. Samprajnata samadhi has two defining characteristics: (1) the consciousness of the meditator becomes identified with the object of meditation, and (2) spontaneous thoughts that are super clear present themselves as immediate knowledge; that is to say, we experience a direct line to intuitive truth. Asamprajnata samadhi is unified consciousness with no cognition, no thought at all. This is a temporary experience of liberation. It is also absolutely necessary to gaining eternal freedom. Each occurrence of samadhi does a little more to burn away our karma and to undo our samskara, eventually allowing us to see and reflect unfiltered reality, Purusha.

That's the gist of chapter one. Of course, there's more to it. Any overview is going to reflect the priorities of the person writing it. To know what's really there, you'll have to read it.

Sadhana Pada

Sadhana means spiritual practice. A good deal of the second pada is devoted to Ashtanga Yoga (which is different from the Hatha Yoga practice of Ashtanga Vinyasa Yoga that K. Pattabhi Jois taught in the 20th century). I'm going to save the discussion of Ashtanga

Yoga for the end of this chapter to maintain the flow of ideas about Kriya.

In this pada, we learn about the causes of suffering or affliction. This is key, since yoga is a practical discipline. There is a problem: life is filled with suffering. There is a solution: practice and detachment, abhyasa and vairagya. This part of the *Sutras* explains why life is full of suffering.

Patanjali lists the causes of suffering or afflictions, called **klesha**, as ignorance, I-am-ness, attachment, aversion, and clinging to life. Let's look a little closer at each.

Ignorance: It is the lack of right knowledge that makes us mistake what is fleeting for what is ultimately important. Not understanding that the material world is temporary and that we are part of an eternal spiritual reality is the foundation of all forms of suffering.

I-am-ness: Through our ignorance of what is changing and what is changeless, we think the ego has a reality all its own. We are deluded by the idea of who we think we are. But personality is malleable and does not have an independent reality.

Attachment: We like and want more of those things we find pleasant. The people, activities, and things we love, however, are impermanent and destined to cease to exist at some point. We become attached anyway and suffer when they go away.

Aversion: We dislike and want nothing to do with experiences that are unpleasant. From petty grievances to the truly horrible and traumatic, all are passing. Even the worst is not forever.

Clinging to life: This is a special case of attachment (to life) and aversion (to death). The will to live is instinctual, and Patanjali assures us this is true even for the wise. There is hope, though, that with enough practice and detachment, when the time comes, as it will, we can let go of our existence on this plane gracefully and with lucid, purposeful awareness.

Actions generated from the klesha create karma, which fuels the cycle that results in more suffering. Patanjali tells us that karma is the source of rebirth. As long as we have the seeds created by karma, we keep coming back, we keep suffering the afflictions, we keep making more karma, and around and around we go.

The goal of all yoga is summed up in sutra 16 of the sadhana pada, which says, "What is to be overcome is future sorrow."[4] Through right understanding we overcome ignorance, and by practicing samyama and compassionate detachment, we start to see the difference between what is temporary and what is eternal. With this recognition, we begin to reflect the Sacred, and we start to live spontaneously from a place of freedom.

Vibhuti Pada

Vibhuti means powers, as in paranormal, psychic powers. The vibhuti pada contains a long list of psychic powers yogis might develop and instructions on how to do so. The content of this chapter is often treated in one of three ways: (1) it is skipped over with an eye-roll and an assumed, "Oh, we know better than that now," (2) it is reinterpreted to be symbolic, or (3) it is assumed to happen only on an energetic level in the subtle body. However, yogis have always been known, and often feared, for their phenomenal psychic abilities.

For Patanjali, if it isn't the Self, it's a distraction. So it's not surprising when he tells us that while samyama on different objects leads to psychic powers, we should ignore these effects because they are not Purusha and we can grow attached to them. They are only more prakriti. He then describes just how to acquire no fewer than twenty-five of these powers.

For the most part the equation goes, "Perform samyama on X and you will gain the ability to Y." For example, samyama on the nature of time yields insight into the past and future (clairvoyance). Samyama into another person's perceptions brings knowledge of that person's mind (telepathy). He goes on to explain how to gain the ability to understand "all beings," to know about previous lives, and to suspend perceptibility (become invisible).

Some powers are more practical. Samyama on the virtues of friendliness, compassion, gladness, and equanimity will infuse you with the energies of those virtues. Physically, you can earn phenomenal strength or freedom from thirst and hunger. Knowledge about the solar system, the universe, anatomy, and consciousness are also there for those who will put in the effort.

As if these abilities aren't enough, Patanjali also tells us how to project the energy body, levitate, bilocate, develop a visible aura, and master the elements, by which he may or may not mean psychokinesis.[5] And, after all of that, he talks about gaining the ***mahasiddhis*** or great powers, I guess because those other feats weren't actually great! The mahasiddhis include shrinking to the size of an atom, growing gigantic, transmigration of the soul, and physical indestructibility.

Now, toward the end of the section on powers, Patanjali tells us that samyama on the moments of time brings the wisdom of discernment. That is to say, meditating on this moment, right now, brings knowledge of what is real and what is temporary, knowledge of the difference between Purusha and prakriti, and that is how we overcome ignorance! Knowledge of Purusha, the higher Self, burns away karma, undoes samskara, and cleans the mirror of consciousness so that we may become reflections of the Sacred.

Kaivalya Pada

In Patanjali's framework, ***kaivalya*** is the end goal. In different translations I have seen kaivalya translated as aloneness, isolation, liberation, freedom, and absolute independence. When we have sat long enough, meditated deeply enough, burned through all of our karma, and come to see through the ignorance and into reality, we are on our way to kaivalya. But not quite there yet.

Unlike most of the rest of yogic philosophy, Patanjali's metaphysics is a dualism. Purusha and prakriti, he says, are separate substances. He also says that to reach complete transcendence one must transcend the physical form. This is one of those aspects of the *Sutras* nobody talks about very much. Most yogis I know believe in some sort of ***jivan mukti*** or living enlightenment. Not so for the *Sutras*. Just like in the *Gita*, we have to make one final exit to gain total liberation from the rounds of birth, death, and rebirth. In the *Gita* it is because we cannot merge with God while we are still in our human form. For Patanjali it is because Purusha and prakriti are separate substances.

Feuerstein explains this when he says, "According to the dualistic model of Classical Yoga, [liberation] implies the dropping of the finite body-mind." He goes on,

> For [Patanjali] the yogin's greatest good lies in severing himself completely from the round of Nature (*prakriti*) and abiding merely as the attributeless Self, one among many and, as we must assume, intersecting with all other Selves in eternal infinity.[6]

Again, this is very different from the identity of atman with Brahman in the Jnana Yoga of the Upanishads or the merging of the individual soul with God in Bhakti Yoga. Be that as it may, our topic now is the *Yoga Sutras*, so—onward!

Chapter four is heavy on abstract philosophy. It delves deeply into karma, samskara, and samsara. It talks about the nature of time and forms. There is speculation on the psychology of perception and the nature of existence.

Eventually, in the final few sutras Patanjali gets to the ultimate experience of kaivalya. We are told that when we can distinguish between Purusha and prakriti, between the Self and the created cosmos, a few things happen. One, we stop building up our egos. With right knowledge and the permanent, ongoing discrimination between the real and the temporary, our little self lets go of its fear and therefore of its continuous need to establish and protect itself. Two, the klesha cease to have any effect and we stop creating karma. Our samskara no longer have hold over us. We are free from suffering. And thirdly, we gain clear insight into the nature of events. Each moment is seen for what it is, the result of various causes and effects. We witness the inter-dependence of all things, and we see all of this without being affected by it. The closer we get to being enlightened, the more we see events from outside the flow of cause and effect. Still, as much as we shed our karma and samskara, while we are living in human form the best we can do is become a clear reflection of the Sacred, which is no small potatoes. It is only after we pass on that we reach ultimate liberation in the meta-physics of the *Sutras*.

And that is a ridiculously brief introduction to the Kriya Yoga that Patanjali presents in the *Yoga Sutras*. We now turn to the second type of yoga in the *Sutras*, Ashtanga.

The Eight Limbs

As promised at the beginning of the sadhana pada, we

return now to Ashtanga Yoga. Engaging the eight limbs
of yoga is a life-altering and lifelong process. Yet, they
take up only 35 of the 195 (or 196) sutras. And they are
given very little introduction. Only one verse leads into
the discussion of the eight limbs; it says,

> Through the performance of the limbs of Yoga, and
> with the dwindling of impurity, [there comes about]
> the radiance of wisdom (*jnâna*), [which develops] up
> to the vision of discernment.[7]

Then it dives right in, as do we. The eight limbs are:

1. Yama: moral restrictions
2. Niyama: moral observances
3. Asana: meditation posture
4. Pranayama: breath control
5. Pratyahara: sense withdrawal
6. Dharana: concentration
7. Dhyana: absorption
8. Samadhi: union

written in the Sutras [handwritten marginal note]

As we'll see, the eight limbs follow each other in
order, one and then the next. Before we can sit and turn
inward to meditate, first we must get our moral lives in
order.

Yama

Yoga, as we've seen, is above all a practical discipline,
and the **yama** and **niyama** are no exception. The goal is
to quiet the mind, and when we follow these ethical

principles, we have less occasion to second-guess ourselves, regret decisions, or need to repair social or emotional damage we've created. It's a jump start on inner peace.

The yama cover interpersonal ethical behavior. That is to say, they tell us how to treat one another and maintain social harmony. Each applies not just to action, but to thoughts and speech as well. The five moral restrictions are:

1. *Ahimsa* (ahimsā): nonharming
2. *Satya*: truthfulness
3. *Asteya*: nonstealing
4. *Brahmacharya* (brahmacarya): chastity
5. *Aparigraha*: greedlessness

Let's look at each just a little more closely. Ahimsa has also been translated as nonviolence and compassion. It comes first not by chance but because it is the most important. All of the other virtues are based on ahimsa. Truthfulness and nonstealing are present, as they are universally in moral codes. Brahmacharya originally meant celibacy, but most modern translations have toned this down to chastity for us householder types. Chastity means not being promiscuous when not in a committed relationship and practicing fidelity when in one. Besides greedlessness, aparigraha has also been taken to mean nonpossessiveness and nonhoarding. It's about maintaining the proper detachment from material goods and could be compared to what we call living simply.

For the most part, the yama help us set the stage for spiritual growth by maintaining peace between us and the rest of the world. But we also need to practice them, especially ahimsa and satya, toward ourselves.

Niyama

The niyama are intrapersonal attitudes and actions undertaken in pursuit of maintaining peace internally. They are as follows:

1. *Shaucha* (shauca): cleanliness or purity
2. *Samtosha*: contentment
3. *Tapas*: discipline or austerities
4. *Svadhyaya* (svādhyāya): self-study
5. *Ishvara pranidhana* (Īshvara pranidhāna): devotion to the Lord

Cleanliness as a virtue was a rather novel idea in 200 CE and may have been why yogis had a reputation for being long-lived. These days, with germ theory and frequent showers being part of our enculturation, we can focus on applying shaucha to our mental and physical environments as well as to our bodies. Keeping our lives, calendars, and minds uncluttered frees up the space we need to maintain our practice and the mindset of compassionate detachment.

Apparently contentment has always been hard-won, as its inclusion in this list would indicate. Living in an economy that depends on instilling a sense of lack in us so we will buy, buy, buy certainly doesn't make samtosha any easier. To be content with what we have goes hand in hand with aparigraha and keeping our possessions limited to what we actually need according to our stage of life.

"Tapas," as we've seen, means "heat" and originally referred to extreme spiritual disciplines such as the *pancha-agni* or five fires, wherein the yogi builds four fires, one in each of the cardinal directions, and sits to meditate between them and beneath the fifth fire of the blazing sun. Standing for years, holding one arm overhead until it withers, and fasting for long periods are all traditional types of tapas.

The *Bhagavad Gita* speaks against these kinds of extreme ascetic practices, calling them ostentatious and pointing out that they ignore that the Sacred dwells in the body. It instead replaces these acts of mortification with mental austerities such as serenity, silence, and self-restraint.[8]

This is one of those instances when it would be really nice to have a commentary from Patanjali's time. He includes tapas as part of Kriya Yoga and Ashtanga Yoga, but we don't really know if he meant the hardcore kind of physical tapas or not. Modern translations seem to be content with defining tapas as commitment to spiritual discipline.

Svadhyaya translates as self-study and, for as long as anyone can remember, has included studying and reciting sacred texts. Studying, contemplating, and memorizing traditional wisdom literature spurs the type of introspection that leads to spiritual growth. It can tell you where you are as well as where you're headed. Study is also useful training in concentration and ego suspension. As it is with any type of flow experience, when we are deeply involved in study, the chatter from our little self subsides.

Ishvara pranidhana adds an element of bhakti to Ashtanga Yoga to go along with the Karma Yoga of compassionate detachment and the Jnana Yoga of study and meditation. We've seen that for Patanjali, Ishvara is a special Self among all interconnected and coinciding Selves, the only one who is untouched by prakriti. Devotion to Ishvara or to an ishta devata is a reminder of that for which we work—to see clearly, to know truth, to be Self.

Sitting and Breathing

With our social lives and inner landscape squared away, we can sit and begin to still the mind. After yama and niyama, the next limb is asana. Originally, "asana" meant "seat." Then it came to refer to a raised platform used specifically as a seat for meditation. In the time of Patanjali, it meant the meditation posture itself. So, the oft quoted sutra, *"sthira sukham asanam,"* or "Posture should be steady and comfortable,"[9] at the time it was written had nothing to do with downward dog or crow pose. It meant we should adopt a sitting position that is easy to maintain for the duration of our practice of pranayama, pratyahara, and samyama.

Pranayama, the next limb, comes from two roots: "prana," meaning "life energy," and "ayama," meaning "to extend." How this came to mean breath control practices is that early on, like Upanishadic early on, seekers noticed that our lives are intimately intertwined with our breath. Life starts with our first inhale at birth and ends with our last exhale at death. The author of the *Amrita Nada Bindu Upanishad* even went to great lengths to calculate the number of breaths we take throughout one cycle of day and night. (That number is 113,180 exhalations and inhalations.[10])

At some point, the idea dawned that the slower we breathe, the longer we live. And, while we have quite a few different kinds of pranayama now thanks to Hatha Yoga, for Patanjali there was one goal—to suspend the breath, as we see in this sutra: "With effort relaxing, the flow of inhalation and exhalation can be brought to a standstill; this is called breath regulation."[11]

Next on the list of limbs comes pratyahara, often called sense withdrawal. This is the necessary step of purposefully removing our attention from our senses. Pranayama helps get the process started as our awareness becomes narrowed to the experience of breathing. We continue to build pratyahara in the next limb, dharana, along with developing single-pointed concentration.

The final three limbs constitute the process of samyama, which was defined earlier in this chapter. To briefly recap, in dharana we do our best to concentrate our attention on an object of meditation. But interruptions happen and we have to keeping letting go of other thoughts and sensations and coming back to the focus of our meditation. Dhyana occurs when the interruptions cease and we become completely absorbed in the practice. Dhyana is effortless. And samadhi happens when the separation between the meditator and the object of meditation disappears and there is unitive consciousness.

To briefly sum up, the eight limbs cover the moral (yama, niyama), physical (asana, pranayama), and psychological or psycho-spiritual (pratyahara, dharana, dhyana, samadhi) aspects of yogic practice.

The Future of the Sutras

If pressed to summarize the message of the *Yoga Sutras* in one sentence, it would be this: the goal of yoga is to still the mind through practice and detachment. The rest, as they say, is commentary.

As we'll see in the next chapter, Patanjali's *Yoga Sutras* comes to define the philosophical school of yoga. Not too much will be made of there being two different approaches to the spiritual path in the same text. And indeed, Kriya and Ashtanga are not irreconcilable. Of the two, Ashtanga Yoga will have the most impact on Hatha Yoga, which keeps the practices but trades in the dualist philosophy for tantric nondualism. And much, much later, Ashtanga Yoga will be labeled Raja Yoga by the Neo-Vedantists who bring yoga to America. "Raja" means "royal," and so the eight limbs come to be called the royal road to liberation.

In American yoga, no other text comes close to being as revered as the *Yoga Sutras*. It's a densely packed piece of wisdom literature which makes it prime fodder for the dozens, if not hundreds, of translations and commentaries that have come into existence in recent times. But we still have eight hundred years to go before Hatha Yoga is even a thing, and another eight hundred before yoga sets foot in the U.S. To see what happens in the meantime, we turn next to the six schools of Hindu philosophy and then take a closer look at the Vedanta school and its champion Shankara.

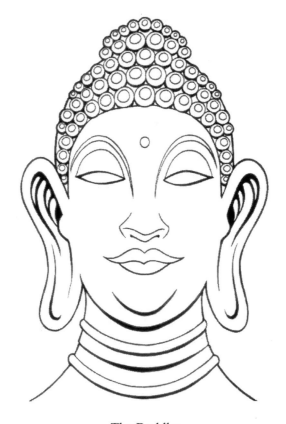

The Buddha

5 VEDANTA AND THE BOY SANNYASIN

Philosophy and religion are not separate things in the Indian tradition like they can be in the West. Explanations of what exists have always been paired with discussions of why; there is no metaphysics without meaning. We saw this in the Vedas, the Upanishads, and the *Yoga Sutras*, and it continues into the next part of our story, in which we look at the six schools of Hindu philosophy, *Vedanta* in particular, and the historical role of one saint or god-man named Shankara.

Six Schools

There are six traditional schools of Hindu philosophy. These schools are referred to as *darshanas* or views, pointing to the Hindu precept that there is one reality and different philosophies are simply different ways of seeing and expressing it. What all of the philosophies have in common is the fundamental tenet that there is an

Absolute, which the Upanishads called Brahman and
Patanjali called Purusha.

Not all of these schools concern yoga, but any story
about the philosophy of yoga needs to give the six
schools at least a passing nod. And, if a student is going
to continue in the study of yoga and Hindu philosophy,
it's especially important to be able to recognize them.
The names of the schools and a brief description of each
follows:

1. *Mimamsa* (mīmāmsā) focuses on the sacrificial
   ritualism of the Vedas.
2. *Vedanta* is based on the Upanishads, the *Brahma
   Sutra*, and the *Bhagavad Gita* and will be further
   explained in this chapter.
3. *Samkhya* (sāmkhya) means "enumeration."
   What it enumerates are the various categories of
   existence. It is similar to Patanjali's yoga in
   holding Purusha and prakriti to be separate
   substances and therefore having a dualistic
   metaphysics. It is different from it in denying
   any role to Ishvara and emphasizing the
   cognitive discipline of discernment (distinguishing the real from unreal, eternal from ephemeral)
   over meditation.
4. *Yoga* in this case refers to the Classical Yoga of
   Patanjali's *Yoga Sutras*.
5. *Vaisheshika* (vaiśeṣika) is an atomistic empirical
   school, meaning it concerns itself with experience that is verifiable through observation and

holds that objects of the physical world are reducible to atoms.

6. *Nyaya* (nyāya) investigates the rules of logic and the art of rhetoric.

The last two schools, Vaisheshika and Nyaya, have little to do with yoga. Samkhya is an important school to become familiar with if you want to go further into studies of the *Bhagavad Gita* or *Yoga Sutras*, as it is interwoven throughout both; however, for the purposes of this overview it's enough to know that it exists and is basically an atheistic form of Jnana Yoga.

Mimamsa, as inquiry into the ritualism of the Vedas, also does not add to our discussion of yoga at this point. But Vedanta does, and it is especially crucial to the iteration of yoga that was exported to the U.S.

These days in the U.S., Patanjali's yoga, Vedanta, and Hatha Yoga are nearly always lumped together, despite some rather major metaphysical differences. This syncretism starts early. In fact it will begin before we leave this chapter. But before we get there, we need to cover the origin and fundamental ideas of Vedanta.

Vedanta

The word "Vedanta" translates as "end of the Vedas," by which is meant the Upanishads. This is because at some point all of the shruti scriptures (the revealed texts, which includes the Vedas, *Samhitas*, *Brahmanas*, *Aranyakas*, and the early Upanishads) became grouped together and just called the Vedas. The Upanishads themselves are, as we saw, a collection of stories, pieces of dialogue, and admonitions from sages about how to find spiritual liberation. They are not, by any means, organized.

The schools of Vedanta started to form between the 4th and 8th centuries CE. Each set out to systematize the ideas of the Upanishads into a coherent worldview. They accepted as their primary texts the early Upanishads, the *Bhagavad Gita*, which has been recognized as an honorary Upanishad for as long as anyone knows, and the *Brahma Sutra*, which might have been the first attempt at systematizing the ideas of the Upanishads, from probably around the 2nd century CE.

All of the Vedantic schools agree on the following principles:

~ Brahman is the all-pervading and eternal cause of the universe.
~ Every person possesses an atman or individual soul.
~ Knowledge (jnana) is a central and indispensable part of the process of gaining liberation from samsara.

These Vedantic ideas—Brahman, atman, and jnana—will come to be some of the most important in all of Hinduism. Later we'll see how, when the 18th century Unitarians and 19th century Transcendentalists begin the American interaction with yoga, it is through Vedanta. And when Vivekananda comes to America in the late 19th century, it will be Vedanta that he brings with him.

Ever since these initial encounters, Vedanta has played a pivotal role in American yoga.

Advaita Vedanta

There are a number of different schools within Vedanta. (That number varies from three to eight depending on who's writing.) And each school has its own interpretation of how to best systematize the ideas put forward in the Upanishads. That is to say, each uses the concepts from those early texts to explain how Brahman and atman conjoin, how the material world exists, and what happens upon liberation. The oldest and most influential of these schools is *Advaita Vedanta*. "**Advaita**" means "not two," or nondual, and refers to its central premise that Brahman and atman are completely identical. According to this school:

~   Brahman is the Absolute.
~   Every person has an atman or individual soul.
~   Brahman and atman are identical.
~   *Vidya* (knowledge) that Brahman and atman are the same leads to liberation.

The practices that lead to vidya are:

Renunciation: both outer and inner. Outer renunciation is detachment from worldly objects and inner is detachment from the ego personality.
Study: svadhyaya is taken by Vedanta to be the study of sacred texts and one's self.

Discrimination: constant awareness of the difference between the eternal and the temporary, between the Absolute and everything else.

Meditation on the mahavakyas (great sayings): introduced in the chapter on the Forest Dwellers, the mahavakya are as follows:

~   Wisdom is Brahman.
~   Atman is Brahman.
~   Thou art That.
~   I am Brahman.

Direct experience (*anubhava*): this comes after a tremendous amount of study and might be thought of as "realization" or a direct experience of what all the stuff that's been studied really means. This is when it all comes together and we really know—not just that we're able to repeat the words, but that we experience the truth of the teachings.

One more key concept to take with us is that it is with Vedanta that Brahman becomes defined as pure consciousness. Okay, so what does it mean that Brahman is consciousness? Consciousness is notoriously difficult to define. At a fundamental level, it is *awareness*, whether that is the self-awareness of a higher primate, the ability of a flower to track the sun, or the quantum entanglement that allows two particles to synchronize regardless of the distance between them. This force, according to the Advaita Vedantists, is Brahman and pervades all that exists. The emergence of this idea in Vedanta was likely the result of interaction with Buddhist ideas.[1]

Buddhist Interlude

I know I promised a linear journey through time, but we need to go back a bit and learn just a few essential tenets of Buddhism to understand the next part of our story. Ready? Here goes no-thing! (That'll be funny in a minute.) (I hope!)

Siddartha Gautama, the Buddha, lived in north-eastern India during the 6th or 5th century BCE. So, that was after the epics but before Patanjali. He was a sannyasin who, after a whole lot of study and brutally intense austerities, finally reached enlightenment through meditation.

The word the Buddha used for enlightenment or liberation from samsara was **nirvana**, which literally means "blown out." This word, "nirvana," had been used before in the Upanishads to mean the same thing as moksha. But there is a difference between the Upanishadic and Buddhist uses of the term. The Upanishads teach that upon transcending conditioned existence we will realize that our individual soul, or atman, is identical with the ground of being, Brahman. The Buddha found no such atman in his experience. Instead he found emptiness, no-thing. And this, he said, was complete freedom, nirvana. Emptiness and **anatman** (anātman), or no-self, are central philosophical components of Buddhism.

The Buddha traveled around northern India for forty-five years, teaching these fundamental principles as well as the Four Noble Truths and the Noble Eightfold Path. Briefly, the Four Noble Truths are (1) life is full of suffering; (2) suffering is caused by desire or craving; (3) desire can be overcome; and (4) the way to overcome desire and suffering is the Noble Eightfold Path, which includes right view, right intention, right speech, right action, right livelihood, right effort, right mindfulness, and right concentration. An underlying truth in the Buddhist worldview is that all sentient beings are equal, karmically speaking, which means that cultivating harmlessness or an attitude of compassion is of supreme importance.

Buddhist doctrine is far too vast for us to cover in any meaningful way here. What's important to take with us are its central principles of emptiness, anatman, and compassion.

The Buddha's message was well received and his ideas spread rapidly. As with any religion that takes root, institutions had to be created, and the Buddha himself ended up having to deal with things like the social structure of the community and specific ethical and metaphysical questions. In many ways, this gave Buddhism a strong foundation as a religious and cultural system.

After the Buddha passed, his wisdom and social institutions continued to thrive. People in the lowest castes and outcastes were especially attracted to the Buddhist rejection of the varnas. In the 3rd century BCE, Emperor Ashoka, who ruled over almost the entire Indian subcontinent, made Buddhism the state religion. In other words, Buddhism became a very big deal and widely replaced traditional Hindu practices.

Okay, with this knowledge of the impact of Buddhism on the religious history of India, we can now turn to the life and ideas of Shankara, who is generally accepted as having revived Hinduism and stemmed the Buddhist tide.

Shankara

Back now to Advaita Vedanta. While as a school it has been around since circa the 2nd century CE, it found its most important historical champion six hundred years later in the figure of Shankara.

Shankara was, it is traditionally acknowledged, an intellectual and spiritual prodigy who shifted the current of religion in India. What we know about his early life comes more from legend than from historical documents, but we can be pretty sure he was born in the late 8th century in the southern state of Kerala to a family of the brahmin caste.

The story goes that from toddlerhood Shankara wanted to take sannyasa and devote himself to the spiritual life. Of course, his parents were not having it. His father passed on when Shankara was five years old, leaving just him and his mother.

One day, when Shankara was eight, he and his mother were bathing in the river near their village. She had gotten out and was resting on the shore when a crocodile took hold of Shankara's leg.

His mother ran to help, holding his arms and pulling him toward her, but the crocodile would not let go. In this moment of what could have been his death, Shankara begged his mother to let him take sannyasa. As soon as she relented, the crocodile released the boy and disappeared under the water. From that moment on, Shankara lived the life of a wandering mendicant, devoted to his own and others' spiritual liberation. He trained first in the Classical Yoga of Patanjali and then in Advaita Vedanta.

In Shankara's time, the religious scene in India was diverse to the point of being chaotic. There were Vedic fundamentalists performing sacrificial rituals by the letter but not the spirit of the law. There were sectarians who claimed their god as the best and only. Tantra was just starting to gain ground, which we will talk about in our next chapter. And, as we just saw, Buddhism was pervasive. Shankara is widely credited with having clarified and strengthened the philosophical positions of Advaita Vedanta and with having brought the various strands of Hinduism together. He was a charismatic speaker, a prodigious writer, a gifted organizer, and a realized yogin. He is remembered as one of the most important figures in the history of Hinduism. He died when he was only thirty-two.

Shankara and Buddhism

The spread of Buddhism and its emphasis on harmlessness and the karmic equality of all sentient beings did help curtail the bloodier sacrifices that were still being practiced by Vedic priests and coming into being in a few tantric sects. But Shankara saw Buddhism as ultimately nihilistic due to its doctrine of anatman.

For Shankara, the major difference between Hinduism and Buddhism was one of "ontology," or what each posits was the essence of being. Hinduism, he said, has a substance ontology. It claims that underlying all the changing surfaces of the material world is an unchanging, permanent entity—Brahman. Another way to think about this is to say that, according to Hinduism, this world is a pattern of impermanent events, made by several different threads woven together to create the sensate world. If you were to pull on one thread, the whole thing would unravel and underneath it all you'd find the Absolute, Brahman. But Buddhism, he said, has a process ontology. It also claims that this world is impermanent and subject to constant change. The difference is, in Buddhism, if you pull on the thread, the whole thing will unravel and reveal nothing at all. This is, of course, diametrically opposed to the fundamental premise of Vedanta, which is that Brahman is the Absolute.

Shankara spent a lot of time refining, explaining, and popularizing the doctrines of Vedanta in order to persuade people away from Buddhism and back to what he saw as the true Indian religion. We'll turn now to the specifics of Shankara's teachings and see just what he said about ethics, metaphysics, and how to reach samadhi.

Ethics

For Shankara, the first steps toward liberation are ethical and practical. Just like in Ashtanga Yoga, we must begin by cleaning up our act; we must morally purify our inner

landscape. The following quotation delineating the
virtues necessary to liberation, as well as all the rest of
the quotations in this chapter, is from Shankara's treatise
The Crest-jewel of Discrimination, as interpreted by
Swami Prabhavananda and Christopher Isherwood. In it
Shankara tells us,

> If you really desire liberation, hold the objects of
> sense-enjoyment at a distance, like poison; and keep
> drinking in with delight such virtues as contentment,
> compassion, forgiveness, straight-forwardness, tran-
> quility and self-control, as if they were nectar.[2]

After becoming established in our ethical lives, then
the work consists of devotion, contemplation, and meditation. The intention is to take control of the senses and
thoughts in order to deconstruct the ego personality.
According to Shankara:

> These are the first steps toward union with
> Brahman—control of speech, refusal to accept
> unnecessary gifts, abandonment of worldly ambi-
> tions and desires, continuous devotion to Brahman.
>
> Be devoted to Brahman and you will be able to
> control your senses. Control your senses and you
> will gain mastery over your mind. Master your
> mind, and the sense of ego will be dissolved. In this
> manner the yogi achieves an unbroken realization of
> the joy of Brahman. Therefore let the seeker strive to
> give his heart to Brahman.[3]

To put this into the Sanskrit we're becoming more familiar with, bhakti, pratyahara, and dhyana lead to samadhi.

Maya

Shankara's emphasis on detachment, distance, and renunciation is consistent with Advaita Vedanta's metaphysical claim that there is only Brahman and what we experience in this world is an illusion created by a force called *maya*. Maya acts through the gunas, which we met previously. To refresh, the gunas are tamas, rajas, and sattva, or inertia, dynamism, and lucidity, respectively.

As a concept, maya has been around since the Vedas, where it meant the power of a deity to create an illusion a human would believe. In the Upanishads it came to mean the sense of illusion where the world is not what it seems. As we see in the next passage, everything in this world of ours is the result of the creative action of maya.

There are the body, the sense-organs, the vital force [prana], the mind, the ego and all their functions, the objects of enjoyment, pleasures and all other kinds of experience, the gross and subtle elements—in short, the whole objective universe, and Maya which is its cause. None of these is the Atman.

You must know that Maya and all its effects—from the cosmic intellect down to the gross body—are other than the Atman. All are unreal, like a mirage in the desert.[4]

Learning to discriminate between what is maya and what is atman or Brahman, words Shankara uses interchangeably, is primary to our goal of being released from samsara.

Karma

In Shankara's formulation of Advaita Vedanta, Brahman is an impersonal force acting through maya and the gunas. Brahman simply metes out what we interpret as fortune and misfortune as determined by the karma of our previous actions. There is no "good" or "bad" in the things that happen to us. Indeed, even in our decisions there are only *avidya* and *vidya*—ignorance and wisdom—in that some decisions move us further from or closer to knowledge of Brahman. And the "fortune" and "misfortune" we may experience, when seen from the perspective of the atman, are equally opportunities to break some connection we have to maya and the material world.

Ishvara

Shankara recognized the difficulty of grasping such an abstract concept as the nondual atman-Brahman, which he also referred to as the one without a second, the self-existent reality, the witness, eternal consciousness, and the Supreme Being. But even with these epithets, most people, at least at some stages of life, need a god with characteristics if not a face.

Without compromising his nondual stance, Shankara claimed that Brahman has two forms: *nirguna* or formless Brahman, and *saguna* Brahman or Brahman with qualities (gunas). Saguna Brahman is Ishvara. Another way to say this is Ishvara is Brahman united with maya. It is Ishvara that creates, preserves, and destroys. It is Ishvara behind the many faces the gods take on. Devotion to Ishvara leads to devotion to Brahman and is one of many practices that help purify the mind and prepare a person for anubhava and samadhi.

Ah, back to samadhi.

Samadhi

After all the work, the moral purification, renouncing externally and internally, studying, contemplating, and meditating, we come again to samadhi. Samadhi is the highest state, the one in which a yogi reaches union, ecstasy, bliss. Remember how in the *Yoga Sutras*, Patanjali spoke of two kinds of samadhi: samprajnata and asamprajnata, or samadhi with cognition and without? Well, Vedanta refers to these as *savikalpa* and *nirvikalpa*. Savikalpa samadhi is unified consciousness with an objective focus. In it, one has an object of meditation with which consciousness becomes united. Savikalpa samadhi contains thoughts that appear as direct knowledge. And nirvikalpa samadhi is beyond thought. It is nirvikalpa samadhi that deconstructs our samskara (deep habits of mind) and burns away any karma that has not yet been activated.

According to Shankara:

> It is a hundred times better to reflect on the truth of Brahman than to merely hear about it from the scriptures. And meditation is a hundred thousand times better than reflection. But nirvikalpa samadhi is infinitely best of all.

> In nirvikalpa samadhi—and in no other state—the true nature of Brahman is clearly and definitely revealed.[5]

On the same subject he said:

> The true nature of the Atman is extremely subtle. It cannot be perceived by the gross mind. It must be known in the state of samadhi which can be attained only by those noble souls whose minds are purified and who possess an extraordinary power of spiritual discrimination.[6]

But, it's worth it:

> When the vision of the Atman, the One without a second, is attained through nirvikalpa samadhi, then the knots of the heart's ignorance are loosed completely and forever.[7]

That is to say, according to Advaita Vedanta, a person can achieve living liberation and become a jivan mukti. Those karmic activators that have been set in motion prior to liberation must play out, and for as long as they take to play out, the enlightened person must remain in their physical form. When the karma is finished and the jivan mukti passes on, that soul will not come back. The individual becomes immortal in the sense that they never have to die again.

Shankara's Achievements

Shankara traveled nearly his whole life, making a complete circuit around India three times. He wrote many commentaries, treatises, and books of poetry. He advocated renunciation but was listened to by those of all walks of life. He sought out spiritual leaders and teachers and challenged them to debate, winning many over with the logic of Advaita Vedanta. Shankara worshipped the gods at local temples wherever he went, regardless of the fact that Krishna was his family deity. By doing this, he maintained the oneness of God, irrespective of incarnation, and set sectarianism aside. He outwitted tantrikas and rallied the Indian people around the traditions stemming from the Vedic lineage and away from Buddhism. He established the first *maths* (pronounced "mutts") or monasteries in India, one each in the north, south, east, and west of the country, all of which are still functioning today. He has come to be considered an incarnation of Shiva.

Shankara merged the philosophy of the Upanishads with Patanjali's Classical Yoga and reminded everyone of the higher goals of bhakti, drawing together disparate aspects of Indian spirituality. It is in no small part due to

Shankara that Advaita Vedanta continues to be an important unifying force in Hinduism today and is deeply influential in American yoga. Advaita Vedanta is traditional and rational, and as different as can be from our next topic, the wild and messy Tantra, which developed right alongside it.

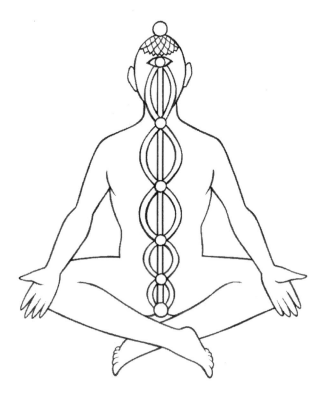

Nadis and Chakras

6 THE TANTRIC EMBRACE OF REALITY

All right dear reader, it's time for Tantra, where things start to get a little wild. A complex and ornate tradition, Tantra Yoga is an amalgamation of ancient goddess worship, traditional magic, and sophisticated psycho-spiritual techniques. Facets of shamanism and the marginalized tribal belief systems overshadowed by Vedic culture resurface in the historical narrative. And it all comes together, creating a paradoxical practice that is at once egalitarian and select. Tantrikas, as people who practice Tantra are called, hold secrecy as fundamental. And Tantra's purposeful inclusion of taboos has brought on vilification since its inception. All of this makes distilling the essence of Tantra a tricky business indeed. But there are some things we do know.

Sometime in the early centuries of the first millennium CE, a small number of low-caste spiritual masters started to organize and systematize what would come to be called Tantra Yoga. Tracing its metaphysics back to the Upanishads, like Advaita Vedanta, Tantra has a non-dual philosophy in which Brahman is the Absolute. But unlike Vedanta, Tantra holds that if there is only one substance, if Brahman truly created and is infused throughout this world, then everything participates in that sacredness. There is nothing that is not divine. Taken into practice, Tantra reclaims everything that the previous yogic traditions bid us denounce, including the material world, the body, and sexuality.

To the enlightened, the Upanishads tell us, there is no difference between clay and gold. Tantra takes it further, saying All is One. For the tantrika, there is no difference between low caste and high, meat and fruit, wine and water. Taboos are only the most prominent way that culture deludes our thinking into false categories, false separateness. In Tantra, every piece of this world is flush with the Sacred and can be used as an instrument toward our spiritual awakening.

The Influence of Caste

Tantra didn't just appear overnight. Elements of it have been around since at least the time when the rishis were discovering the Vedas. It is, in no small way, the religion of all the people the Vedic culture cast out, the tribes that were swallowed up, and the women who were silenced.

Vedic rituals belong to the brahmins. The karma and dharma teachings of the epics speak to the kshatriya caste. And Advaita Vedanta can be seen as a rarified abstract philosophy for those who are ready to entirely detach from this world. But Tantra was created from the religious practices of the common people and the lower castes, who found their spirituality in a cosmology that values everything, without distinction. It is world-embracing.

There is academic debate over whether the first tantric texts, which are also called Tantras, were Buddhist or Hindu. The oldest extant Tantras are Buddhist, but the earliest Hindu Tantras refer to even earlier ones that are now lost. The upshot is that Hindu and Buddhist Tantra developed simultaneously, probably with little regard for the religious labels we use now. Tantra as a cultural movement infiltrated all of the religious paths of India, including Jain and Sikh traditions. Here we will focus solely on the Hindu incarnation, because it is from there that Hatha Yoga, the yoga of the body, was born.

Tantra, like all yoga, is at heart a practical system of spiritual development. Different from other branches of yoga, though, Tantra is indiscriminate. If a method works, it has a place in Tantra. Tantric texts talk about cosmology, metaphysics, yama and niyama, hundreds of deities, goddess worship, elaborate and complex rituals, magic, the subtle body, physical and mental purification, mantras, mudras, yantras, visualization practices, break-ing taboos, and the nature of moksha. And all of these are necessary, they say, because we are in a backward time, when spiritual discipline needs all the help it can get.

Yugas

According to Hindu cosmology, time is cyclical. Upon the birth of the universe, time begins and creation enters the first of four *yugas* or ages. Depending on the source, these ages are either tens of thousands or even millions of years long. Each subsequent age is "darker" than the previous. The ages are the *Krita, Treta (Tretā), Dvapara (Dvāpara)*, and *Kali* Yugas. The Dvapara Yuga is said to have ended when Krishna left the earth at the end of the war in the *Mahabharata*. Which leaves us in the **Kali Yuga**. As it says in the *Mahānirvana Tantra*: "Now the sinful Kali Age is upon them, when Dharma is destroyed, an Age full of evil customs and deceit."[1] Kali is the fierce black-skinned goddess of time, change, and destruction. The word "kali" translates as dark, but a long, long time ago it used to refer to a bad throw of the dice.[2]

In each subsequent age, the weight of virtue versus vice shifts toward vice, from light to dark. In the Krita Yuga, there was only virtue. The texts of that time were the shruti: the Vedas, *Brahmanas*, *Aranyakas*, and Upanishads. And these were enough because people's purity allowed them to find realization through these texts alone. In the Treta Yuga there was one-quarter vice and three-quarters virtue. In this age came the smriti, the texts which were remembered. These include but are not limited to the epics, the Puranas, and the sutras of the various schools of philosophy. The third age, Dvapara, was equally weighted toward vice and virtue. People of this time found their religion in lore and legend. And in the Kali Yuga we face three-quarters vice and one-quarter virtue. We need all the help we can get. The Tantras are written specifically for this age.

At the end of the Kali Yuga, the universe will end. After a period of dormancy lasting 311,040,000,000,000 (that's three hundred and eleven trillion, forty billion) years, the universe will be born once more and the cycle will begin again.[3]

Brahman

Much of what we know about Hindu Tantra comes from translations and commentaries originally published under the name of Arthur Avalon. Avalon, it turns out, was the pseudonym for the duo of Sir John Woodroffe and Atal Behari Ghosh. Woodroffe was a British judge on the Calcutta High Court in the late 1800s and early 1900s, and Ghosh served as Sanskritist and translator for the team. Together they made over twenty Tantras available to the English-speaking world.

And what they tell us is that, in Tantra, Brahman is the supreme, unconditioned Absolute, and just like in Vedanta, Brahman exists in two forms: saguna and nirguna, that is to say with qualities and without. Brahman, says "Avalon" in the *Introduction to Tantra Sastra*, "is embodied in the form of all Devas and Devis, and in the worshipper himself. Its form is that of the universe, and of all things and beings therein."[4] (***Devas*** and ***devis*** are deities; literally, "shining ones.")

Brahman suffuses this world, making every bit of it Sacred. But we miss it, too busy with our profane lives

139

to see that we, our loved ones, the people on the street, every tree and rock and grain of sand are the miraculous incarnation of divinity. To break the hold that ignorance has on us and to facilitate the experience of Brahman, the experience of enlightenment, Tantra takes advantage of every available path. According to the experienced tantrika Shuddhananda Bharati in the preface to the *Tantrarāja Tantra:*

> The Tantra Yoga adapts all the eightfold accessories of the Raja Yoga, takes the best in all systems of Yoga and transcends them in the conquest and enjoyment of Nature. It is a union of the Puruṣa with Prakṛti, conceived as the Universal Mother. There are poses, mudras, breath-controls, concentrations, chants and meditations but more than all these, there is the delight of the conquest of the lower nature by the higher to make life an integral factor of Bliss Divine.[5]

I want to stick with this passage for a minute and shine a light on a few key ideas. First of all, "the eightfold accessories of the Raja Yoga" here refers to the ashtanga or eight limbs in Patanjali's *Yoga Sutras*. This is a rather modern usage of the term, from probably the 19th century on. When it is used in the Hatha Yoga texts we'll cover in the next chapter, Raja Yoga refers to the mental rather than physical spiritual practices.

After that, the next important word in this quotation is "enjoyment." Enjoyment, or ***bhoga***, refers to sensory enjoyment and is an important aspect of Tantra. This sets

Tantra apart from other paths again, in that so far we have been admonished to renounce the enjoyment of sense-objects. A common phrase says that Tantra is both yoga and bhoga.

And finally, when he refers to poses, these are seated meditation postures. Soon enough we will talk about the early asana of Hatha Yoga, but for now asana still means seated posture.

The meaning of the passage, with or without these wriggly details, is that the goal of Tantra is to realize that the material world *is* the spiritual world. Said in the language of various yogic philosophies: Purusha and prakriti are not separate substances; the small self is a manifestation of the higher Self; matter and Spirit are identical; samsara is nirvana; All is One.

The Goddess

One of the most distinguishing characteristics of Tantra is the centrality of the feminine divine to the process of liberation. In cultures around the world, male and female are symbolic of the transcendent and the immanent respectively. Women represent the world of nature. With our monthly cycles in tandem with the moon and tides, with childbearing and breastfeeding, which so obviously tie us to the realm of mammals, this connection isn't a leap. In many, many cultures, rather than being cele-brated, our special connection to the natural world has relegated us to lesser status. But in Tantra, where nature and spirit coincide, and where the physical world is meant to be enjoyed, the feminine in the abstract and women in the flesh are worshipped as the Goddess, the manifest power of the Sacred. The feminine divine appears in Tantra as multiple goddesses, as the creative power of the universe, and in ritual sex.

As we have seen since the beginning of our story, the different faces of the gods and goddesses of India are understood to represent the many facets of the Sacred. And Tantra accepts them all; however, Shiva and Shakti are given pride of place. The Tantras are recorded as conversations between these two deities, and they are incarnated in the subtle body of every human. Energetically speaking, Shakti lives at the base of the spine and takes the form of the kundalini, or serpent power. Shiva resides at the top of the skull or just above. The practices of Tantra (and Hatha Yoga, as we will see in the next chapter), awaken the kundalini, which then rises up the spine connecting Shiva and Shakti.

Shakti means "power," and the goddess Shakti is the creative power of the universe. She is saguna Brahman. The union of Shiva and Shakti represents the union of male and female, matter and Spirit, all pairs of opposites.

Each of the devis is a special manifestation of the Divine Power. Kali, Durga, Tara, Parvati, Sita, Radha, and a hundred other goddesses represent various cosmic forces. Many of the goddesses take on fierce and frightening forms, only to become symbols of comfort and love to their devotees. Through complex, detailed visualization practices, devotees identify with the deities. This kind of practice encourages the experience of embodying the Sacred, of becoming one with the Goddess, joining in union, in yoga, with her.

Panchamakara

Breaking taboos is an important ceremonial aspect of Tantra. This is fully embodied in the ritual of the five *m*'s or *panchamakara* (pancamakāra). Only advanced tantrikas participate in this ritual, which is named after five forbidden substances that all happen to start with the letter *m* in Sanskrit.

~ *Madya*: wine
~ *Mamsa* (māmsa): flesh
~ *Matsya*: fish
~ *Mudra* (mudrā): parched (dry-roasted) grain
~ *Maithuna* (maithunā): intercourse

It's easy to understand why alcohol and the flesh of animals, whether of the land or sea, have been held as taboo, but dry-roasted grain? Apparently it was seen as a consciousness altering aphrodisiac. These first four elements must be consecrated through ritual. Then, as they are consumed, sexual energy is accumulated. The pinnacle of the ceremony is using that energy in the act of sex to awaken the kundalini. Because we live in the Kali Yuga, this ritual is said to be too powerful for most tantrikas, and substitutes such as milk, sugar, and honey are recommended for wine, meat, and fish. And sex is symbolically replaced with meditation on the Goddess.[6]

Some tantric sects choose to practice a literal interpretation of the five *m*'s and other ritual practices of taboo breaking. These sects are said to follow the left-hand path. Those following the right-hand path choose the symbolic interpretation. Either way, the underlying symbolism of disregarding cultural conditioning and overcoming our mental categories is the essence of the practice.

The Subtle Body

Some aspects of Tantra, like the subtle body, mudras, and mantras, are well known to American yogis because they play an important role in Hatha Yoga. This is because, as we will see, Hatha Yoga began as a movement within Tantra. Let's look at these individually.

The idea of the subtle body isn't original to Tantra. We saw it before in the *Taittiriya Upanishad's* discussion of the pancha kosha or five sheaths. What Tantra adds is a thorough description of the prana body. In practice, some people experience this body on a sensory level, and others find it a useful tool on a more metaphorical level.

Prana flows into the body with a baby's first inhale and leaves the body upon our last exhale. And while prana is coterminous with the breath, meaning they happen together, it is not the same as the breath. This can be said for the whole subtle body. It is coterminous with the physical body but not the same thing. And the **chakras** (pronounced with a hard "ch," as in "chair") might be coterminous with our nerve plexuses, but they are something else altogether.

Here's how it works. The subtle body is made of prana, which travels via nadis (channels). There are a lot of these nadis, perhaps hundreds of thousands of them, but we are only going to focus on the three most important ones: the sushumna, the *ida*, and the *pingala*. All three of these travel along the spine.

The sushumna is the central channel. It goes from the base of the spine right up to the crown of the head, from Shakti to Shiva. However, in most of us, the kundalini, which is a special, intense manifestation of sacred creative power, lays coiled at the entrance to this channel. This dormant spiritual energy blocks the flow of prana from entering the sushumna and forces it to take an alternate route, through the ida and pingala.

The ida is associated with the left side of the body, the feminine, and the moon. Sort of like yin. The pingala is associated with the right side, the masculine, and the sun. Sort of like yang.

The ida and the pingala spiral up the outside of the central channel, and where they cross they create pools or eddies of energy called chakras.(See the illustration at the beginning of this chapter.) "Wheel," "vortex," "circle," and "center" are all literal translations of "chakra." The intention behind the many practices of Tantra Yoga (and Hatha Yoga) is to purify the energy body so prana can flow freely through the ida and pingala, then to awaken the kundalini and move the energy into the central channel. Only then can this powerful spiritual energy flow through the sushumna, uniting Shiva and Shakti and bringing on the state of samadhi.

Chakras

According to Woodroffe and Ghosh's translation of the 16th century *Sat Cakra Nirupana* (*Description of the Six Centers*), the chakras are named and located as follows:

~ *Muladhara* (mūlādhāra) / root support: perineum
~ *Svadhistana* (svādhiṣṭhāna) / own base, seat of the self: sacrum
~ *Manipura* (maṇipūra) / city of jewels: navel (solar plexus in some traditions)
~ *Anahata* (anāhata) / unstruck [sound]: heart
~ *Vishuddha* (viśuddha) / purity: throat
~ *Ajna* (ajña) / command: behind and between the eyebrows
~ *Sahasrara* (sahasrāra) / thousand petaled: crown of the head or slightly above it[7]

There are six chakras but seven listed because the sahasrara is not a pool of our own prana but rather a potential site of incoming cosmic energy.

In the *Sat Cakra Nirupana* we are given each center's name, location, and shape; which god, goddess, and animal abide there; and the siddhis or vibhuti a yogi develops when the chakra is sufficiently meditated upon. For example:

By meditating thus on Her who shines within the Mūla Chakra [muladhara], with the lustre of ten million Suns, a man becomes Lord of speech and King among men, and an Adept in all kinds of learning. He becomes ever free from all diseases, and his inmost Spirit becomes full of great gladness. Pure of disposition by his deep and musical words, he serves the foremost of the Devas.[8]

Each ascending chakra earns increasingly greater powers.

Nowadays there are loads of interpretations of chakras and their qualities. They've been assigned everything from psychological traits to planets to gemstones to essential oils. These are all products of the 20th century. There are colors assigned to each chakra, but they do not match up with the rainbow spectrum so often linked to the chakras today. For the curious, they are:

~ Muladhara: golden yellow
~ Svadhistana: vermillion
~ Manipura: the color of a stormy sky
~ Anahata: the color of *bandhūka*, a bright red flower
~ Vishuddha: smoky purple
~ Ajna: white like the moon[9]

The chakras come to fruition in Tantra and carry over into Hatha Yoga. They are an essential aspect of spiritual development in both traditions, since balancing them is fundamental to getting prana to flow freely first through the ida and pingala and then in the sushumna.

Let's look at a few more tools Tantra provides for spiritual growth: mantras, mudras, and yantras.

Mantras

Mantras are sacred sounds and words of power. Their use in spiritual practice is called *japa,* which means repetition. Japa can be spoken out loud, repeatedly softly, recited internally, or written.

Mantras have a long history. The verses of the Vedas are considered mantras, and the sacred syllable Om, as we've seen, has its own Upanishad, the *Mandukya.* Mantras are not arbitrary but rather are sounds discovered by rishis and sages in their deepest meditations and travels to higher states of consciousness.

Some folks these days say mantras are a technique to quiet the mind, to distract us from our incessant mental chatter and bring us to one-pointed concentration. And that they do. Traditionally, however, mantras have been used for different reasons. Some are meant to prevent misfortune or gain good karma. Others are straight up magic. And some embody states of energy or consciousness. Through repetition and samadhi with the mantra, the yogi comes to embody that state, too.

Mantras are regarded as more powerful when they are transmitted by a guru. Since the time of the Vedas, the dynamic of teacher-to-student transmission has been indispensable to yoga. As yoga has been, and still is in some places, an oral tradition, the guru embodies the sacred text. A truly enlightened teacher is able to guide individual students in exactly the way they need. And where mantras are concerned, a guru doesn't only intuitively know which sacred sound is right for the student, but they can activate it, empowering it.

But the guru dynamic didn't translate very well into American yoga, due possibly to our rampant individualism and definitely to the charlatans and sexual predators who have posed as gurus throughout yoga's tenure in the U.S. Since very few of us are going to find liberated souls to be our teachers and transmit mantras to us, does that mean we shouldn't use them or that they won't have the same effect as if they did come from a guru?

On the flip side, mantras are also said to gain efficacy through vast numbers of repetition. Some schools insist it is the sound of the word itself that carries the power, in which case where it comes from might not matter, but proper pronunciation would be essential. Others say it is the concentration on the intention behind the japa that produces the benefits. If any of these are the case, then mantras still have a positive effect regardless of where they come from.

Mudras

Whereas mantras are sacred sounds, mudras are sacred gestures. The word mudra is usually translated as "seal" or "energy seal," and the gestures serve many purposes. They can be used to bring about various states of consciousness. Some people can feel them literally alter their energetic field. There is a whole category of mudras that are therapeutic, encouraging healing on the physical level. Mudras serve a communicative purpose in art, symbolizing the qualities of deities and sages. And they are used in ritual worship and meditation.

On this final front, Feuerstein describes how complex tantric worship involving mudras can be:

> Thus according to the *Mantra-Yoga-Samhitā*, nineteen seals are necessary in the worship of Vishnu, ten for Shiva and the Goddess Tripurā-Sundharī, nine for Durgā, seven for Ganesha, five for Tārā, four for Sarasvatī, two for Rāma and Parashu-Rāma, and only one for Lakshmī.[10]

Today there are two mudras that are ubiquitous in American yoga. One is the anjali or *namaste* (namastē) mudra, in which the hands are brought to touch with the palms and fingers pressed gently together. This mudra represents honoring or showing respect. The other is the jnana or wisdom mudra, wherein the tip of the thumb and forefinger of the same hand are brought to lightly touch. Here the thumb represents the Sacred and the index finger represents the individual soul. In this mudra, the Self and the self form an unending circuit.

As we will see in the next chapter, in Hatha Yoga many mudras engage the whole body and not just the hands.

Yantras

And finally, a brief word about **yantras**. Yantras are specific geometric designs that play an important role in tantric visualization and meditation. These complex shapes carry vast symbolism and represent both a deity and the yogi's own ego, showing the correlation between macrocosm and microcosm. The forms are memorized by the adherent, and visualized in a specific order, from outside to inside. Then the image is deconstructed or erased in reverse, thereby evaporating the practitioner's small self and promoting the experience of union with nirguna Brahman, which is the end goal of all of these practices.

One Mountain, Many Paths

Mudras, mantras, and yantras are just a few of the many spiritual exercises of Tantra Yoga. It is a sumptuous, ornate, practice-centered tradition that holds the material world and the spiritual world as equally sacred. It brings together elements from all of the previous yogas and, according to Woodroffe and Ghosh, all of these practices are, as the saying goes, paths up the same mountain:

> Whether yoga is spoken of as the union of [Shakti] with [Shiva], or the union of the individual soul (jīvātmā) with the Supreme Soul (paramātma), or as the state of mind in which all outward thought is suppressed, or as the controlling or suppression of the thinking faculty (cittavṛtti), or as the union of the moon and the sun (Idā and Pingalā), . . . , the meaning and the end are in each case the same.[11]

The meaning and end are to experience union, yoga. Or, as Pierre Bernard, America's first Hatha Yoga teacher and a tantrika through and through, would have it, "The material world is lit to its atoms with the spark of God.

The key to the mystery of life—if you care to know—is this unrealized unity."[12]

The Tide of History

Between the 8th and 14th centuries CE, central power in northern India disintegrated and was replaced by multiple kingdoms and vassal states. This political situation led to religious regionalism and rivalry. During this time, various sectarian versions of Tantra developed. From then on there have been separate tantric sects devoted to Shiva, Vishnu, Shakti, and Buddhist deities. It was also during this time that Hatha Yoga developed from many sources, not the least of which was one of these tantric sect devoted to Shiva.

Shall we?

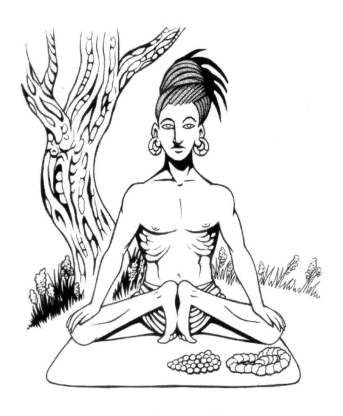

Hatha Yogin in Gorakshasana

7 THE YOGA OF THE BODY

Thank all the gods and goddesses! We have *finally* made it to Hatha Yoga! Welcome to the beginning of all the different kinds of body-centered yoga.

Before we dive in, another little note about pronunciation. There is no "th" sound in Sanskrit like in the word "the." It always sounds like the "th" in "hothouse." Phonetically, hatha can look like "hə-tə" or "huh-tuh."

Okay, with that out of the way—"hatha" means "forceful" and refers to the intensity of this branch of yoga. Hatha Yoga blends elements from Ashtanga Yoga, Advaita Vedanta, and Tantra, as well as alchemy, and then adds its own unique physical practices. Its original proponents came from the Siddha Movement that began in Tantra around the turn of the first millennium.

We've seen the word "siddhi" before; it means perfection or power, especially supernatural power. A *siddha* is a person who has realized siddhis. The Siddha Movement was based on reverence for a group of eighty-four men and women who had achieved moksha as well as siddhis; they were called the mahasiddhas. The prefix "maha" means "great." The mahasiddhas were venerated as deified human beings (and they still are in the tantric form of Buddhism). The mahasiddhas did not identify solely as Hindu or Buddhist but spanned the line between them.

Physical perfection and immortality were central concerns of the Siddha Movement, especially to the two mahasiddhas who would found the Shaivite *Natha* (Nātha) lineage and create Hatha Yoga. These were Matsyendra and Goraksha.

Matsyendra

The historical Matsyendra (often called Matsyendranath) lived in the early 10th century. He was the first Hatha yogin and had many students, including Goraksha (Gorakshanath), who by all accounts was a charismatic teacher and a miracle worker and played a crucial role in the dissemination of Hatha Yoga.

There are many legends explaining how Matsyendra learned the secrets of Hatha Yoga from Shiva, the Lord of Yoga. Here is one version.

Shiva decided to share the teachings of Hatha Yoga with his wife, the goddess Parvati; however, these powerful teachings needed to remain closely held secrets. He could only speak them aloud in a safe place, where no one would overhear. So Shiva and Parvati went to the ocean floor where they created a giant air dome in which to hold these sacred lessons.

Years earlier, in the world of humans, a child had been born under terribly inauspicious astrological signs. This child, who would become Matsyendra, was cast into the ocean at birth. He was swallowed whole by a giant fish, and inside this fish he grew to be a man.

The stories of Shiva and Matsyendra meet up when Matsyendra, inside his fish, came across Shiva teaching Parvati inside their bubble under the sea. Matsyendra stayed nearby, listening and learning. Parvati eventually became bored. (Goddess devotees say this was because she already knew everything about Hatha Yoga and was just humoring her husband!) As Parvati's eyes glazed over, Shiva said, "Fine! Is there no one listening to me?"

"I am listening," said Matsyendra from his fish.

So Shiva continued to teach Matsyendra the secrets of Hatha Yoga. Matsyendra stayed in the fish practicing what he had learned for another twelve years, and then his fish was caught and sliced open. He emerged, a fully realized yogin.

Matsyendra means "Lord of the Fishes."

The Body in Hatha Yoga

Hatha Yoga starts with the tantric idea that the created world is sacred and then focuses the practical emphasis squarely on the body. Previous to Tantra, the body was mostly seen as something to be overcome. In *The Crest-jewel of Discrimination,* Shankara echoes the disgust we saw in the *Maitrayania Upanishad* back in chapter 2 when he says, "This body, which is made up of skin, flesh, blood, arteries, veins, fat, marrow and bone, is full of waste matter and filth. It deserves our contempt."[1] And later he reiterates, "Detach yourself completely from this covering, the body, which is sluggish and foul. Having done this, never think of it again. To remember one's own vomit is merely disgusting."[2] I think he makes his stance quite clear there.

And could that body-bashing perspective be more different than this verse from the 17th century siddha Bhogar?

Time was when I despised the body;
but then I saw the God within.
The body, I realized, is the Lord's temple;
And so I began preserving it with care infinite.[3]

In Hatha Yoga, the body is the aspect of the Sacred we inhabit and for which we are responsible. The physical practices of Hatha Yoga are meant to keep the body healthy and strong so it can endure long periods of meditation and the trial of kundalini awakening. Some texts, such as the *Yoga Bija*, said to have been written by Goraksha himself, and the *Yoga Shikhā Upanishad*, from the 13th century, even refer to the alchemical creation of a "diamond body" that is "adamantine" and vibrates much faster than regular matter, to the point where it can change shape and disappear from view.[4]

Without a doubt, the body becomes an important tool in the process of liberation for Hatha Yoga, but it isn't the only one.

The Practices of Hatha Yoga

Three texts are considered to be classics of Hatha Yoga. They are the *Hatha Yoga Pradipika* from the 14th century; the *Siva Samhita* from either the late 15th or late 17th century; and the *Gheranda Samhita* from the 17th century, which is the most complete. Most of what follows comes from these three works.

The *Gheranda Samhita* tells us that Hatha Yoga is composed of seven practices. These are:

~   Shat karma: "six actions" of purification
    (sometimes called *shat kriyas*)
~   Asana: postures
~   Mudras: seals (which here includes bandhas or
    energy locks)
~   Pratyahara: sense withdrawal
~   Pranayama: breath control
~   Dhyana: meditation
~   Samadhi: union

As we can see, these practices are not only about the body but include the higher mental practices, too. In fact, the practices of Hatha Yoga run the gamut from physical to mental to pure being. To break this down, on the physical side there are the shat karma, asana, mudras, and bandhas; spanning the physical and the mental are pratyahara and pranayama; dhyana is a state of consciousness; and samadhi is pure being.

Dhyana and samadhi are referred to as Raja Yoga in Hatha Yoga texts. For instance, the *Siva Samhita* defines

Raja Yoga as meditation to the point where the "modi-fications of the mind are suspended."[5] And later it admonishes that "the *hathayoga* cannot be obtained without the *rajayoga*, nor can the *rajayoga* be obtained without the *hathayoga*."[6]

While practitioners of the more conservative and traditional types of yoga, like Vedanta, considered Tantra and especially Hatha Yoga to be crude and of lower status, Hatha yogins have always viewed their approach as more complete than other paths because it includes the entire body-mind.

Let's check out these seven practices of Hatha Yoga individually.

Shat Karma

Cleanliness was important long before Hatha Yoga, as we saw with shaucha in the niyamas of Ashtanga Yoga. But the shat karma take cleanliness and physical purifi-cation to a whole new level, striving to purify the body inside and out. The *Gheranda Samhita* lists the shat karma as the following:

~ *Dhauti* (dhautī): cleansing, including cleaning the teeth, tongue, and sinuses; the throat; and the anus.
~ *Basti*: a water or air enema with no equipment!
~ *Neti* (netī): running a thread through a nostril and out the mouth. Today this is often performed by pouring water from a neti pot in one nostril and allowing it to drain out of the other.

~ *Nauli* (naulī): rolling the abdominal muscles to massage the internal organs.

~ *Trataka* (trāṭaka): gazing steadily at a small object until tears flow.

~ *Kapalabhati* (kapālabhāti): skull shining breath, a breathing technique of short, forceful exhales.

The *Hatha Yoga Pradipika* makes it clear that not everyone needs to perform the shat karma; they are only necessary for people in poor health. Some of the purification techniques could be dangerous and should only be attempted under the supervision of an experienced teacher.

Asana

Before Hatha Yoga, "asana" referred only to meditation postures. The yoga of the body adopted and expanded upon these seated poses. The asana of Hatha Yoga serve many purposes: they heal and strengthen the body; they build discipline and concentration; and they facilitate the flow of prana in the energy body. While there are now hundreds of asana, the *Gheranda Samhita,* which has the most to say on the subject of the three classic texts, describes only thirty-two. Twenty of those thirty-two are seated, and only one is standing.

In the following list, I've divided these asana by type, giving the Sanskrit name and English translation. If the posture has a different modern name, I've added that at the end of each entry. I've italicized those for which there is no matching posture in modern postural practice. Many of those that are italicized will sound familiar, but the postures as they are described in the classic texts are different than those in contemporary sources. I encourage the interested reader to check out James Mallinson's translation of the *Gheranda Samhita*, which includes photographs of each asana as well as some of the mudras.

Seated

~ Siddhasana (siddhāsana): perfected posture

~ Padmasana (padmāsana): lotus posture

~ Bhadrasana (bhadrāsana): fortunate posture (today often called baddha konasana [koṇāsana] / bound angle posture)

~ *Muktasana (muktāsana): freedom posture*

~ Vajrasana (vajrāsana): diamond posture (today also known as virasana [vīrāsana] / hero posture)

~ *Svastikasana (svastikāsana): auspicious posture*

~ Simhasana (siṁhāsana): lion posture

~ *Gomukhasana (gomukhāsana): cow face posture*

~ Virasana: hero posture (description matches the legs of our contemporary bharadvajasana [bharadvājāsana] II / Bharadvaja's posture)

~ *Dhanurasana (dhanurāsana): bow posture*

~ *Guptasana (guptāsana): secret posture*

~ Matsyendrasana (matsyendrāsana): Lord of the Fishes posture

~ Gorakshasana (gorakṣāsana): cowherd posture

~ Paschimottanasana (paschimottānāsana): intense stretch of the west posture

~ Sankatasana (sankatāsana): contracted posture (legs of contemporary gomukhasana / cow face posture)

~ *Kurmasana (kūrmāsana): tortoise posture*

~ *Mandukasana (maṇḍukāsana): frog posture*

~ *Uttanamandukasana (uttānamaṇḍukāsana): raised frog posture*

~ *Garudasana (garuḍāsana): eagle posture*

~ *Vrishasana (vrishāsana): bull posture*

~ Yogasana (yogāsana): union posture

Prone

~ Shalabhasana (śalabhāsana): locust posture

~ Makarasana (makarāsana): sea monster posture (sometimes called crocodile posture today)

~ Ushtrasana (uṣṭrāsana): camel posture (similar to present day dhanurasana / bow posture)

~ Bhujangasana (bhujangāsana): cobra posture

Supine

~ Shavasana (śavāsana) / mritasana (mritāsana): corpse posture

~ Matsyasana (matsyāsana): fish posture

~ Uttanakurmasana (uttānakūrmāsana): raised tortoise posture (description matches what we call garbha pindasana [pindāsana] / embryo in the womb posture)

Arm balances

~ Mayurasana (mayūrāsana): peacock posture

~ Kukkutasana (kukkuṭāsana): rooster posture

Squatting
~ Utkatasana (utkaṭāsana): fierce posture
(description matches what we call malasana
[malāsana] / garland posture)

Standing
~ Vrikshasana (vṛkṣāsana): tree posture

Pretty different from what a Hatha Yoga class looks like these days! No warriors or downward facing dogs or sun salutations. Plus, it's likely that proficiency in these postures was measured by one's ability to hold them for a very long time. As we'll see in Theos Bernard's report on his personal experience with traditional Hatha Yoga, he was taught that the goal was to hold certain postures for three hours!

While the asana do have strengthening, healing, and preventive qualities, they aren't just for the benefit of the physical body. When performed correctly, the postures allow prana to flow freely through the nadis of the subtle body. Especially important is balancing the prana in the ida and pingala, which spiral up around the central channel of the spine, the sushumna. As we saw in the previous chapter, the unrestricted flow of the life force balances the chakras, or energy vortices where nadis cross. Energetically, the goal of asana is to bring the prana into the sushumna and awaken the kundalini. When the kundalini circulates in the sushumna, it brings about samadhi.

On an esoteric level, "ha" and "tha" stand for sun and moon, and we saw previously that the pingala represents the sun and the ida the moon. And that is why Hatha Yoga is said to be the union of the sun and moon.

Mudras

Mudras are seals that help control the flow of prana. While today people are usually referring to hand gestures when they talk about mudras, there are several seals that involve the full body. Some of the positions we might recognize as asana are actually listed as mudras in the old texts.

The bandhas are sometimes considered mudras and sometimes listed on their own. "Bandha" means "lock" and refers to locking prana within the torso, again, controlling the flow of energy. There are three bandhas:

- ~ *Mula* (mūla) *bandha*: contracting the anal sphincter and lifting the pelvic floor
- ~ *Uddiyana* (uḍḍīyāna) *bandha*: pulling the abdomen in and up
- ~ *Jalandhara* (jālandhara) *bandha*: contracting the throat by pulling the chin inward

Performing all three at once is called *maha-bandha*.

Now that we have the bandhas under our belts, here are some of the mudras and their shapes according to the *Gheranda Samhita:*

- ~ *Mahamudra:* press the left heel to the perineum and extend the right leg. Take hold of the right big toe with the first two fingers of both hands.

Inhale, take jalandhara bandha, and hold.
Release the chin lock and exhale slowly.

~ *Nabho mudra:* flip the tongue upward and let it
rest on the roof of the mouth, moving it toward
the soft palate, and restrain the breath. This can
be done at any time.

~ *Khechari mudra:* lengthen the tongue by "milk-
ing" it and cutting back the frenum underneath
little by little, until it can be rolled back into the
esophageal passage. The actual mudra is performed by blocking the nostrils with the tongue
from inside the airway.

~ *Viparitakarani:* place the head on the ground
and raise the legs into head stand. (Some schools
interpret this as reverse posture, which is a
modified shoulder stand.)

~ *Yoni mudra:* In siddhasana, press the thumbs
over the ears, the index fingers over the eyes, the
middle fingers up against the nostrils, the ring
fingers on the upper lip, and the pinky fingers on
the lower lip.

~ *Vajroli mudra:* place the hands on the ground
and raise the legs in hand stand.

Pratyahara

Pratyahara refers to turning our attention inward and
letting the passing sights, sounds, smells, and so on go
unnoticed or at least unattended. Sense withdrawal is
usually facilitated by turning the mind toward an object
of concentration; this can be a small object, a mantra, a

visualization, or the breath. It is the first step in building concentration.

A present-day formulation of the idea behind pratyahara can be found in Mihaly Csikszentmihalyi's (it's pronounced cheeks-sent-me-hi) description of the psychological state of "flow." In the flow state, our focus becomes absorbed in an activity to the point that sensory information doesn't make an impression. For example, some situations that can induce a flow state include reading a great story, creating art, studying, video games, sports, and puzzles. When we experience flow, time can appear to change, moments might seem to go by in slow motion while hours disappear. In pratyahara, we induce the flow state in the act of concentration or contemplation.[7]

Pranayama

As we have seen, pranayama are breathing exercises that help to grow the life force within us. Different prana-yama techniques have different effects. Some are heating and some are cooling. Some slow the central nervous system and some enervate it. The goal of many of these breathing exercises is to lengthen the duration of **kumbhaka** or retention of breath, just as we saw in the *Yoga Sutras*.

The *Hatha Yoga Pradipika* and *Gheranda Samhita* both describe various kinds of alternate nostril breathing as preparatory to pranayama practice. Breathing through one nostril at a time is said to open both the ida and pingala evenly, preparing the prana body for the work to come. Here are the types of pranayama according to both of these texts:

~ *Suryabheda kumbhaka:* Breathe in strongly through the right nostril. Retain the breath and take jalandhara bandha. Hold for as long as "the perspiration does not burst out from the tips of the nails and the roots of the hair."[8] Then, release the bandha and exhale slowly.

~ *Ujjayi*: The *Gheranda Samhita* says to perform ujjayi, first breathe in through the nose, hold the air in the mouth, then exhale through the mouth and take jalandhara bandha. The *Hatha Yoga Pradipika*, on the other hand, says that the throat should be closed and "air should be drawn in such a way that it goes touching from the throat to the chest, and making noise while passing,"[9] which is how the practice is usually taught today.

~ *Sitali* (sītalī): Open and purse the lips, breath in through the mouth with "the tongue thrown out." Hold for a brief time, and then exhale through the nostrils. The *Hatha Yoga Pradipika* also describes *sitkari* (sītkārī), a similar breathing technique where the tongue is kept "between the lips."[10]

~ *Bhastrika* (bhastrikā): Treating the lungs as if they are bellows, breathe in slowly through the nose and then exhale quickly. After twenty rounds, retain the breath.

~ *Bhramari* (bhrāmarī): The *Hatha Yoga Pradi-pika* says to inhale strongly, making a noise like a wasp, and exhale slowly making the same noise. The *Gheranda Samhita* calls bhramari pranayama the "beetle droning kum-bhaka"; however, it then goes on to explain it as a practice of covering the ears and becoming aware of various internal sounds.[11]

~ *Murchha* (mūrchā): Here we have another where the texts might be interpreted as differing. The *Gheranda Samhita* says of this one, "having performed Kumbhaka with comfort, let him withdraw the mind from all objects and fix it in the space between the two eyebrows. This causes fainting of the mind, and gives happiness."[12] And the *Hatha Yoga Pradipika* describes it by saying "closing the passages with Jālandhar Bandha firmly at the end of Pūraka (inhalation), and expelling the air slowly, is called mūrchā, from its causing the mind to swoon and giving comfort."[13]

~ *Plavini* (plāvinī): The final pranayama in the *Hatha Yoga Pradipika* is the plavini or floating pranayama. It is described like this: "the inside of the body is filled to its utmost with air, the body floats on the deepest water, like the leaf of a lotus."[14]

~ *Kevali* (kevalī): This is the final pranayama in the *Gheranda Samhita*, which first explains that all people continuously and unconsciously make the sound of "sah" as they inhale and "ham" as they exhale. Together, these sounds make "so' ham," which means "I am that," or "hamsa," which means "Great Swan."[15] In kevali pranayama, the yogi makes this sound and meaning conscious and alters the number of breaths per minute, adding retentions.

The purposes of pranayama include increasing concentration, lengthening the life span, and maneuvering the prana toward awakening the kundalini.

Dhyana

The *Hatha Yoga Pradipika* tells us that Shiva taught 2.5 million methods of meditation.[16] And the *Gheranda Samhita* describes several of them, including visualizations similar to those in the Tantras. It also lists several possible objects of contemplation, including the guru or a god or goddess, Brahman and atman, or various facets of the subtle body, including chakras and the kundalini. There is also a section dedicated to contemplation of the light within the prana body.

In the chapter on the *Yoga Sutras*, we learned that dharana, or concentration, is what we are usually doing in "meditation," when thoughts continue to intrude and we make the effort to keep our attention focused. And then dhyana refers specifically to the state of consciousness that occurs when the rest of the world has receded and there is only our subjective awareness (the "I") and the object of concentration. The Hatha Yoga texts combine dharana and dhyana, using dhyana to refer to both states.

Samadhi

Beyond the state of meditation is samadhi, union. The ultimate samadhi is union with Brahman, which can occur with cognitive content or without, just like Brahman can have qualities (saguna) or not (nirguna). In Tantra and Hatha Yoga, it is said that whenever samadhi occurs, the kundalini is flowing in the sushumna. While some extremely advanced realized sages can control samadhi, at first it is spontaneous and unpredictable. It doesn't always happen during meditation, though it can. But it can also come on out of the blue. Besides the yogi's dedicated practice, the grace of a guru can also induce the state of samadhi.

At the end of the *Gheranda Samhita*, we hear the by now familiar message of enlightenment. In samadhi the yogi realizes: "I am Brahman and nothing else. I am Brahman alone and do not suffer. My form is truth, consciousness, and bliss. I am eternally free. I abide in my own nature."[17] "Truth, consciousness, and bliss" come from the Sanskrit "satchitananda," which is also sometimes translated at "being, consciousness, and bliss."

Through the experience of its true nature, the free soul comes to recognize all living things and the whole world to be part of the same and only Self, and through samadhi escapes suffering and samsara. For the Hatha yogin there is absolutely the possibility of becoming a jivan mukti and experiencing liberation in this lifetime.

And when and if the body dies or transubstantiates into light, there will be no rebirth for the liberated atman.

The *Hatha Yoga Pradipika* states plainly that this is the goal: "All the methods of Hatha are meant for gaining success in the Raja Yoga; for, the man who is well established in the Raja Yoga overcomes death."[18] And with its last verse it warns us that practice is essential. Yoga is something to be done, not just talked about:

> As long as the Prāna does not enter and flow in the middle channel . . . ; as long as the mind does not assume the form of Brahma[n] without any effort in contemplation, so long all the talk of knowledge and wisdom is merely the nonsensical babbling of a mad man.[19]

How to Practice Hatha Yoga

There is a fascinating passage in Pancham Sihn's 1914 translation of the *Hatha Yoga Pradipika* that gives us a look into a day in the life of a yogi. While Tantra provided a spiritual path for anyone, including householders, in Hatha Yoga the pendulum has swung back toward living the removed life of a sannyasin. The grammar of this translation is not smooth, but I could not find another that included this passage.[20] I have forgone the use of [sic] to avoid making the passage even more difficult to read. I have also included a few explanatory words in brackets. Every-thing in parentheses is from the translated text.

I am going to describe the procedure of the practice of Yoga, in order that Yogis may succeed. A wise man should leave his bed in the Usā Kāla (i.e., at the peep of dawn or 4 o'clock) in the morning.

Remembering his guru over his head, and his desired deity in his heart, after answering the calls of nature, and cleaning his mouth, he should apply Bhasma (ashes).

In a clean spot, clean room and charming ground, he should spread a soft āsana (cloth for sitting on). Having seated on it and remembering, in his mind his guru and his God.

Having extolled the place and the time and taking up the vow thus: "To day by the grace of God, I will perform Prānāyāmas with āsanas for gaining samādhi (trance) and its fruits." He should salute the infinite Deva, Lord of the Nāgas [Shiva], to ensure success in the āsanas (postures).

Salutations to the Lord of the Nāgas, who is adorned with thousands of heads, set with brilliant jewels (*Manis*), and who has sustained the whole universe, nourishes it, and is infinite. After this he should begin his exercise of āsana and when fatigued, he should practise Śava āsana. Should there be no fatigue, he should not practise it.

Before Kumbhaka, he should perform Viparīta Karnī mudra, in order that he may be able to perform Jālandhar bandha comfortably.

Sipping a little water, he should begin the exercise of Prānāyāma, after saluting Yogindras [the Gods of Yoga], as described in the Karma Parana [Kūrma Purana], in the words of Śiva.

Such as "Saluting Yogindras and their disciples and gurū Vināyaka [Ganesha], the Yogī should unite with me with composed mind."

While practising, he should sit with Siddhāsana, and having performed bandha and Kumbhaka, should begin with 10 Prānāyāmas the first day, and go on increasing 5 daily.

With composed mind 80 Kumbhaka should be performed at a time; beginning first with the Chandra (the left nostril) and then sūrya (the right nostril).

This has been spoken of by wise men as Anuloma and Viloma. Having practised Sūrya Bhedan [single nostril breathing beginning on the right], with bandhas (the wise) should practise Ujjāyī and then Sītkārī, Śītalī, and Bhastrikā, he may practice others or not.

He should practise mudras properly, as instructed by his guru. Then sitting with Padmāsana, he should hear anāhata nāda [unmade sound] attentively.

He should resign the fruits of all his practice reverently to God, and, on rising on the completion of the practice, a warm bath should be taken.

The bath should bring all the daily duties briefly to an end.

At noon also a little rest should be taken at the end of the exercise, and then food should be taken. . . .

After taking food he should read books treating of salvation, or hear Purānas and repeat the name of God.

In the evening the exercise should be begun after finishing sandyhā [a Vedic religious ritual], as before, beginning the practice ghatikā or one hour before the sun sets.

Evening sandhyā should always be performed after practice, and Hatha Yoga should be practised at midnight.[21]

Okay, so just get up early, purify the body, and pray; then do asana, alternate nostril breathing for eighty rounds, four other pranayamas, and meditate on the unstruck sound. Then take a bath. Repeat the process at noon, followed by studying the sacred texts. Repeat at dusk, adding some Vedic prayers. And repeat again at midnight.

No wonder you have to be a sannyasin—there isn't any time left for work, family, or anything else for that matter! Add to this the admonition from the same text that:

> The Yogī should practise Hatha Yoga in a small room, situated in a solitary place, being 4 cubits [approx. 6.5'] square, and free from stones, fire, water, disturbances of all kinds, and in a country where justice is properly administered, where good people live, and food can be obtained easily and plentifully.[22]

In other words, celibacy, isolation, and intense, life-long commitment were part and parcel of being a yogi.

Time and Change

These are the teachings of Hatha Yoga as it developed between 1000 and 1500 CE. They were held in utmost secrecy, passed on orally from guru to student, until the movement was threatened. With the coming of the Mughals in the early 16th century, the need must have arisen to preserve the tradition in writing. And indeed, beginning with the Mughal dynasty and continuing through the occupation by the East India Company and the British Raj, Hatha Yoga faced redefinition, discrimination, and drastic change.

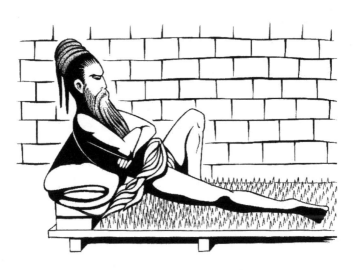

A Yogi on a Bed of Nails

8 THE IMPACT OF EMPIRES

Hold on to your hats, or your mats, as the case may be! This chapter covers a couple of raucous centuries in the history of yoga. We'll begin in the 16th century by looking at how the practices of Hatha Yoga were co-opted toward violent ends during the Mughal era. Then, in the 17th and 18th centuries, the British move in and drastically change the landscape. And finally we check out the early American encounters with yoga and end up at the beginning of the 20th century.

Ascetic Warriors

Around the same time the oldest extant Hatha Yoga texts were written, the practices they espoused were being co-opted for a far different purpose than spiritual liberation. This part of our story begins in the 1500s, when most of northern India fell to the Mughals, an invading force from the area that is now Uzbekistan (northeast of

Pakistan and Afghanistan, extending past the Aral Sea). By the early 1700s, nearly all of India was part of the Mughal Empire.

During this era, it became a common practice for some young Indian men to leave their villages and seek their fortunes as ascetic mercenaries. They dressed and trained as yogis, but their intention was to earn and/or steal enough wealth to return home, marry, and start a family.

These men lived in groups that were either nomadic or resided in ashrams or maths. Besides their Hatha Yoga practice, they trained in martial arts and weaponry, too. This explains why yogis from this time are often portrayed carrying spears, bows and arrows, swords and shields, and metal disks with sharpened edges called chakras.

Some scholars interpret the existence of these warrior yogis in terms of class warfare: the poor, young, indigenous men versus the wealthy imperialist Mughals. And their main target was indeed the Mughals, especially along trade routes, but at times they clashed violently with other similar Hindu, Sikh, and Muslim groups. The tradition of the ascetic warrior continued on for generations. Interested readers can find the full fascinating story in Judanath Sarkar's classic text from 1930, *A History of Dasnami Naga Sannyasis* and William R. Pinch's much more recent *Warrior Ascetics and Indian Empires*.

The East India Company

We need to take a brief aside to set the stage for the British to enter the scene, as everything from this point forward happens either with them or because of them.

This part of our story begins with the British East India Company (EIC). In 1600, the EIC was given a government-sanctioned monopoly on trade between England and all of the countries on the Indian Ocean. Their first ship landed on Indian shores in 1608, and in 1615 they were given permission from the Mughal rulers to set up a coastal "factory" in Surat. Factories, named after the "factor," as the official in charge was called, functioned as offices and warehouses. The most important exports were spices, indigo, raw silk, and cotton textiles.

Eventually the EIC set up more factories both along the coast and inland. Over time the areas around these factories became thriving urban centers for trade, manufacturing, and education—all financially dependent on the EIC. The cities of Madras, Bombay, and Calcutta, which are now renamed Chennai, Mumbai, and Kolkata, all grew around the economic stimulus of the EIC.

Between 1700 and 1750, the Mughal Empire went into financial crisis due to invasions by Persia and Afghanistan leading to expensive wars; farmers moving off their land because of high tax rates and opportunities in cities; and indigenous rebellions. All of these factors led to widespread decentralization, resulting in independent provinces and a power vacancy that the EIC stepped in to fill with its hierarchical organization, modern communications, and army.

And what an army it was. To protect their trade routes and factories, often from the very ascetic mercenaries we were just talking about, the EIC built up a powerful force. It was made up of English officers with well-paid Indians filling out the ranks. The British also sent whole regiments to assist them.

By 1765 the EIC was the largest territorial power in India and levied taxes in the regions it controlled. In 1784 the British parliament began placing regulations over how the EIC could function in its governing roles. And by the end of the 18th century, all of India was under British law. Finally, in 1858 the British government took over all governing functions from the EIC, and India officially became part of the British Empire.

That is a very brief version of the story of how the English came to rule India, first through economics and then through politics. Granted, it is a woefully inadequate version from a human rights perspective, but it is enough for us to move along with the story of yoga.

Warrior Yogis and the British Raj

Now we can loop back a bit and pick up again with the warrior yogis. When the EIC showed up in the 17th century, the militant yogis (and they were called yogis or *jogis*) naturally had a new target. Of course, not all yogis were warriors, but the warrior yogis were the only ones with whom the EIC and the British Raj were concerned. After decades of violent clashes, in 1773 the Governor-

General of India, Warren Hastings, made it illegal to wander naked or to carry a weapon near trade routes; in sum, he made it illegal to be a yogi.[1]

Once this ban was in place, many of these mercenaries, now deprived of their ill-gotten gains, ended up in cities with no means of support. Talk about *personae non gratae!* Among Indians, yogis were casteless in a caste-based society, literally outcasts. The English, for their part, were moving into the Victorian era, and yogis clothed only in loincloths and dreadlocks, if at all, were certain to offend by their very presence. Plus, these particular yogis were known to be violent.

This is how many of these former militants ended up on the streets, now mendicants relying on handouts for their sustenance. Some became buskers—street hustlers, magicians, and contortionists, performing torturous austerities for money. In the early 1800s, street yogis and *fakirs,* their Muslim equivalent, became a popular subject for the new medium of photography. Pictures from this time show yogis enduring various types of extreme tapas. Some have held their arms up above their heads for so long the limbs have become withered and useless. Others wear large metal grids welded around their necks in a way that makes it impossible for them to lie down. Still more are shown piercing their cheeks or chests with long needles and bleeding very little. The most iconic image of this era may be the bed of nails.

There was a mix of sideshow theatrics with sincere spiritual commitment going on. The most radical practices made for the most popular pictures, so that is what became representative of yoga to the West. Within the yogic tradition, however, the deep current of renunciation and quiet meditation in the pursuit of spiritual liberation still prevailed.

Even if the warrior ascetics weren't truly representative of the spirit of yoga (ahimsa anyone?), they are of historical significance for at least three reasons. First, with the warrior yogis we see the first time Hatha Yoga was taught and learned in groups. Second, the migration to cities explains the transition between yoga as something done only in isolation to yoga in public. In other words, yoga was no longer a secret. And finally, the image of the yogi as emaciated beggar, seen by Indians and English alike as a blight upon society, played an important role in how Hatha Yoga would become reformulated in the early decades of the 1900s. Consciously or not, the founders of the Hatha Yoga renaissance distanced themselves from the image of the warrior ascetic and the street yogi.

The British Influence

British rule influenced Indian culture in a great number of ways. Three in particular stand out as key threads in our narrative: translations, education, and starvation.

Translations

Many of the early government representatives felt that to better understand and control the Indian populace, it was imperative to come to grips with the Hindu religion. In their efforts to describe what we've seen is a tremendously amorphous cultural entity, they would put forth observations and designations of what "Hindu" meant, and native Hindus would then either confirm or refute these ideas. This process eventually led to the defintion(s) of Hinduism that we have now.[2]

The interest the colonizers took in Hinduism also led to the creation of schools for the study of Sanskrit and the translation of many sacred texts into English. Among these early translations were the Upanishads, the *Bhagavad Gita*, and the *Yoga Sutras*. These translations would make their way across the world to fascinate European Romanticists and philosophers as well as early New England Unitarians and the Transcendentalists.

Education

Perhaps the most far-reaching decision on behalf of the British was to introduce English-style education for Indians, through which they created an Indian middle class of English-speaking professional and service-sector workers. Along with whole-hearted belief in rationalism, science, and technology, the British very purposefully incorporated Western values in their pedagogy, including ideals such as liberty and equality. Can you see where this is going? Two major developments came about because of this program of instruction, both of which had unintended consequences and neither of which worked in favor of the British.

First, English became a common language among groups who previously didn't have one. Indians from the furthest reaches of the country could now communicate with each other, and this widespread communication meant that nationalism could take root on a whole new scale. Second was the spread of the idea of fundamental human rights. At first, this led to indigenous reform movements that supported the Raj in the abolition of female infanticide, child marriage, polygamy, and the caste system. But the values of liberty and equality cannot apply for some and not for others, and eventually these also fed the independence movement.

Starvation

While the EIC had moved in to export goods only India could provide, with the spread of English power came an increased demand for resources dedicated to trade. By instituting programs in which the best lands were used to produce export crops like tea, coffee, opium, and cotton, the British induced famine in India. Not enough land was left to feed the people, and millions died. Famine, while also stoking the fires of the independence movement, was a motivator in the lives of two of the most influential voices in the early American encounters with yoga, Raja Ram Mohan Roy and Swami Vivekananda, both of whom we will meet before this chapter is out.

Early American Interactions with Hinduism

Now, from this point on our story no longer moves in a straight line, if it ever did. The world is industrializing; intercontinental shipping and travel are not fast but also not uncommon; Indians are Western educated, and Westerners are receiving communications and translations from India. The influence between East and West is not just bi-directional, it's becoming web-like.

THE IMPACT OF EMPIRES

America enters stage left.

Cotton Mather

More than fifty years before the United States was even a thing, the religious discussion between America and India started. And it started the way you might expect, as more of a monologue than a dialogue.

The first recorded American encounter with the spiritual paths of India came through no less a figure than the fire-and-brimstone spewing epitome of New England Puritanism that was Cotton Mather. When he wasn't whipping up Salem's witchcraft frenzy, Mather found time to correspond with Danish missionaries in India. In response to them, he wrote *India Christiana* (1721), detailing his proposal for converting Hindus to Christianity. [3]

Unitarianism

Actual reflection on Hinduism by an American had to await the advent of the academic field of comparative religions. So it wasn't until three-quarters of a century after Mather that Joseph Priestley, now best known as the guy who discovered oxygen as a chemical element, wrote *A Comparison of the Ancient Institutions of Moses with those of the Hindoos and Other Ancient Nations* (1799).[4] Priestley's approach blatantly set out to prove the superiority of Christianity, but at this point in history, did you really expect anything else? Nope, not really.

Which is what makes the next development so interesting.

Priestley was a Unitarian, but unlike Priestley many early American Unitarians dug Eastern philosophy and religion. Before we go on, we need to know a little bit about **Unitarianism** because it is an important part of the story.

Unitarians are so called because they are monotheists, believing there is one God. Some would say they are radically monotheistic, since they go so far as to say that other Christian denominations are not monotheists but rather are Trinitarians because, you know, the Trinity.

Two other characteristics of Unitarians set the stage for them to be receptive to yogic ideas. One is their conception of God as a power or force rather than as a personal deity. The other is their fervent belief in the individual. Unitarians believe each person carries within them a "divine spark" and that no one should ever be coerced into any religion or practice. Each individual should be free to determine their own spiritual path.

In the second half of the 18th century, when the first translations of Indian holy books started turning up in New England, Unitarians mined them for treasures. They found plenty of ideas that resonated with their own beliefs. It's not much of a stretch from a God characterized as an impersonal power or force to Brahman, or from atman to a divine spark. Plus, they probably identified with the idea in the *Bhagavad Gita* that different people are suited to different spiritual paths.

Taking a step back to get a wider perspective, we see that the first Americans to consider yogic ideas as a viable addition to their spiritual life were primarily interested in an individualistic type of spirituality; they weren't looking to adapt rituals or social structures. And they only had access to texts. In other words, the early American Unitarians were exposed to the philosophical substratum of yogic ideas and not to the lived tradition. This abstraction was perpetuated by interactions between Unitarians and a very important Indian named Ram Mohan Roy.

Ram Mohan Roy

Roy is called the "Father of Modern India." He was English-educated and deeply influenced by Unitarianism. He was also a nationalist and a tireless advocate for social reform. Roy petitioned the English to end the famine they had created. He promoted the study of the English language and English-style education in the sciences. He fought for the abolition of what he saw as barbaric and superstitious practices among his fellow Hindus, such as caste, polygamy, child marriage, and *sati* (in which widows were burnt alive on their husbands' funeral pyres). He disdained "idol worship" and promoted what he considered to be a return to the ethics and spirituality of the Upanishads, which he interpreted as a monotheism consistent with the Unitarian view of Christianity.

Roy worked for and with Englishmen most of his life. In 1821 he collaborated with the Baptist missionary William Adam to translate the New Testament into Bengali. During this time Adam converted to Unitarianism. That same year, he and Roy cofounded the Calcutta

Unitarian Committee, even though Roy never converted to Christianity. After seven years of working together, Roy and Adam had an irreparable disagreement over which languages were appropriate for liturgical use. Adam wanted to use Bengali in religious services, but Roy believed only Sanskrit, Persian, and English were fit to be used as sacred tongues. So, in 1828, Roy pulled his support from the Committee. Later that year he founded the highly influential religious reform group, Brahmo Samaj.

Neo-Vedanta

Roy and the Brahmo Samaj were staunch advocates of what has come to be called **Neo-Vedanta**. Neo-Vedanta is a reformulation of Advaita Vedanta in response to colonialism and modernity. It bears the stamp of values Roy and his contemporaries picked up through their English education, values such as egalitarianism and tolerance, rationalism and empiricism. It was also influenced by the liberal Christian esotericism of Unitarianism.

Neo-Vedanta shares the fundamental beliefs of Vedanta: Brahman is the Absolute; each individual has an atman; and liberation is found through the realization of their identical nature. Setting it apart from Advaita Vedanta, Neo-Vedanta doesn't require renouncing the world and is accessible to everyone, regardless of stage or station in life. Also different is that it places personal experience as primary, even above the wisdom found in the sacred texts.

Like Advaita Vedanta, Neo-Vedanta champions Hindu unity, which in this new setting took on a nationalistic tone. But the importance of Hindu unity didn't preempt Neo-Vedanta's further tenet that all faiths are equal. The description of the spiritual quest in terms of many paths up the same mountain was expanded to include all religions, not just all schools of yoga. And with Neo-Vedanta we see a return to the idea of loka samgraha (world gathering). That is to say, for Neo-Vedanta working for the good of the world is an essential part of spiritual life. This is big. Not only does Neo-Vedanta not advocate renouncing the world, it strongly advocates working on behalf of humankind.

Because Roy translated many ancient Indian texts into English, he had a guiding hand in how yogic ideas were presented to the West and especially back to Unitarians. Thus we witness the continuation of this web of influence, this time connecting English education, devout Neo-Vedanta Hindu popularizers, and English and American spiritual seekers: Roy was influenced through his English education and by the Unitarians; his ideas would have a strong effect on Indian culture; and the books he translated would help shape the next generation of Unitarians, some of whom became the Transcendentalists.

An important point to reiterate here is that Roy was influenced by Unitarians who had already begun with an abstracted idea of yoga. Then he helped formulate and propagate Neo-Vedanta, which some would say abstracted it even further from its cultural bearings. Or maybe yoga was just becoming reconciled to *new* cultural bearings, informed by modernity and its adulation of rationalism, science, and equality. However you look at it, the yoga being shuttled back and forth between America and India was mostly a type of Jnana Yoga with elements of Karma.

Transcendentalism

Transcendentalism was the first great American philosophical and literary movement. It lasted from around 1830 to the 1880s. The Transcendentalists were a loosely allied group of New England thinkers and writers, who believed fervently in individualism and idealism. Idealism is the metaphysical stance that the world of ideas is more real or fundamental than the material world.

The writings of the Transcendentalists have been in print since the movement started. Their ideas influenced authors such as Nathaniel Hawthorne, Herman Melville, and Walt Whitman, and philosophers like Henry James, William James, John Dewey, and George Santayana. The ideology of the Transcendentalists forms part of the foundation of American culture.

The Transcendentalists themselves were influenced by thinkers of their day, and none more so than the Unitarians. Like the Unitarians (and Neo-Vedanta), the Transcendentalists believed in one God and that each of us has a piece of God within.

But the Transcendentalists considered Unitarianism a bit vanilla. They were after intense and personal spiritual experiences. They wanted first-hand knowledge of the Sacred and gave priority to the intuitive and spiritual over experiences based in the senses or in reason. In that way they show the influence of another important cultural force of the time, Romanticism. And, to continue the multi-directionality of influence, the Romantics had themselves been inspired by early translations of the *Bhagavad Gita* and, even more so, the Upanishads.

The Transcendentalists magnified and glorified both the individualism and the yogic ideas they inherited from Romanticism and Unitarianism, and none of them to a greater extent than its superstars, Ralph Waldo Emerson and Henry David Thoreau.

Emerson, the Intellectual Omnivore

Emerson's father was a Unitarian minister, as was Emerson himself for a brief time. However, his father passed on when Emerson was still young, and it was another Unitarian, his aunt Mary Moody, who first introduced him to the sacred texts of India.

Four years after leaving the Unitarian Church over misgivings about public prayer and serving Communion, Emerson attended the first ever official Transcendental Club meeting in 1836. At the core of Transcendentalism was the idea that through nonconformity a person might escape cultural conditioning and have a true, unmediated experience of God. In this way Transcendentalism took on the goal of all yogas—to decondition the psyche and experience the unmediated Absolute.

Emerson was an intellectual omnivore, and the translations he was familiar with of the Upanishads, the *Bhagavad Gita*, and other Eastern texts must have both informed his ideas and helped him describe his thoughts on nature and humankind. We see this at work in his poem "Brahma," published in 1856 or '57.

Brahma

If the red slayer think he slays,
    Or if the slain think he is slain,
They know not well the subtle ways
    I keep, and pass, and turn again.

Far or forgot to me is near,
    Shadow and sunlight are the same,
The vanished gods to me appear,
    And one to me are shame and fame.

They reckon ill who leave me out;
    When me they fly, I am the wings;
I am the doubter and the doubt,
    And I the hymn the Brahmin sings.

The strong gods pine for my abode,
    And pine in vain the sacred Seven;
But thou, meek lover of the good!
    Find me, and turn thy back on heaven.[5]

And for this beautiful poem, Emerson received much more ridicule than reward. These ideas were so far removed from everyday life in the 1800s as to be indecipherable to most folks. From then on, he kept his more overtly Eastern ideas to his letters and journals;

although, if you're familiar with the premises of yogic thought, their influence can be felt throughout his writings.

Still and again, Emerson's incorporation of yogic ideas was an intellectual one. He adopted abstracted, rarified ideas from texts and never experienced the lived tradition. Henry David Thoreau, on the other hand, at least experimented with the idea of *being* a yogi.

Thoreau, the Sannyasin of Walden Pond

Thoreau was another Transcendentalist who learned not to inundate his readership with obscure Eastern ideas. After including several references to the *Bhagavad Gita* and other sacred books in *A Week on the Concord and Merrimack Rivers*, he was accused of both blasphemy *and* being too preachy, which is a pretty interesting combination of criticisms.

But the yogic approach to life is never far from the surface of Thoreau's work. During his retreat to Walden Pond, he kept the *Gita* on his bedside table, where it captured his imagination:

In the morning I bathe my intellect in the stupendous and cosmogonal philosophy of the Bhagvat Geeta, since whose composition years of the gods have elapsed, and in comparison with which our modern world and its literature seem puny and trivial; and I doubt if that philosophy is not to be referred to a previous state of existence, so remote is its sublimity from our conceptions. I lay down the book and go to my well for water, and lo! there I meet the servant of the Bramin, priest of Brahma and Vishnu and Indra, who still sits in his temple on the Ganges reading the Vedas, or dwells at the root of a tree with his crust and water jug. I meet his servant come to draw water for his master, and our buckets as it were grate together in the same well. The pure Walden water is mingled with the sacred water of the Ganges.[6]

In a letter to his friend and admirer, H. G. O. Blake, Thoreau discusses his experiences of stillness and contemplation, saying: "Depend up on it that, rude and careless as I am, I would fain practice the yoga faith-fully. . . . To some extent, and at rare intervals, even I am a yogi."[7]

Where's the Bhakti?

It is striking, as Christopher L. Walton points out in "Unitarianism and Early American Interest in Hindu-ism," that Bhakti Yoga, the yoga of divine love, was quite absent from the early American adoption of yoga. Karma they accepted; contemplation, meditation, aus-terities, the unity of Brahman—check. Devotion to a personal deity? Nothing doing.[8]

Was this somehow because of the Unitarian rejection of a personal God? Was it due to that same bias in translations that came from Ram Mohan Roy and other Anglo-educated Indians? Would a personal deity have threatened the Romantic view of individualism and free will? Whatever the cause, the yoga of Tran-scendentalism was, for the most part, a text-based, intellectual abstraction of the spiritual paths of India and a far cry from how Hindus actually lived their religion.

In the long run, the Transcendentalists' ideas, peppered as they were with yogic insights, have been significant throughout yoga's integration with American culture. Transcendentalism directly influenced the New Thought movement, which we will see in a moment in turn influenced the first truly successful Hindu missionary to the U.S., Swami Vivekananda. And much later the Beat poets would claim the Transcendentalists as a major influence. Mohandas Gandhi took his ideas for nonviolent resistance in no small part from Thoreau's essay, "Civil Disobedience," and Martin Luther King, Jr., took these ideas from Gandhi, continuing the interplay between the strands of the web.

However, while Transcendentalism has been highly influential in the history of American ideas, in the late 1880s, when its stars faded out, yoga itself hadn't exactly caught on. For the most part, the few people who knew about it saw it as very much "other" and not as something to incorporate into their daily lives.

But before the century was over, Swami Vivekananda would come and let everyone know that yoga is something you *do*, not just something to read about.

Swami Vivekananda

At the end of the 19th century, a Hindu popularizer and social activist, who was looking for help combatting the famine in India, brought a version of yoga already informed by Western values to America. He had no problem finding people who were receptive to his message.

Swami Vivekananda came to America in 1893 to speak at the Parliament of Religions at the Chicago World's Fair. While his mission was to raise money for his starving countrymen, he ended up being one of the most significant figures in the story of yoga in the modern world, East and West.

The swami embodied a combination of the mysticism of his guru, Ramakrishna, and the modern social reform views of the Brahmo Samaj. He was also English-educated and counted the Transcendentalists among his spiritual influences. He was an ideal ambassador.

Right out of the gate, Vivekananda framed his proposition as trading the spiritual advancements of India for the material goods of the U.S. Playing to the pre-existing fascination with Eastern mysticism among certain segments of the American population, Vivekananda's work relied on and solidified the stereotypes of the spiritual East and materialistic West.

What He Taught

Vivekananda's guru, Ramakrishna, was a jivan mukti whose spiritual path included Tantra and Kali worship, Vaishnava bhakti, and Neo-Vedanta. The Brahmo Samaj, to which Vivekananda previously belonged, also promoted Neo-Vedanta. Two ideas in particular that came from the Brahmo Samaj, one from Ram Mohan Roy's era and one from after his time, were hugely influential in how Vivekananda talked about yoga. The first is that he said *anyone* can practice yoga. With its many paths, he said, yoga can accommodate anyone and everyone. The second was how he defined these paths. Just like the Brahmo Samaj, Vivekananda said there are four types of yoga: Karma, Bhakti, Jnana, and Raja.

In Hatha Yoga, Raja Yoga referred to the higher mental practices as opposed to the physical practices. In the terminology of Neo-Vedanta it's different; here Raja Yoga means the Classical Yoga of Patanjali's *Yoga Sutras*, especially the eight limbs.

The four yogas method of categorization became the customary way in the U.S. and in India to discuss the different yogic paths. And while all the yogas have the same goal, and all paths lead up the same mountain, according to Vivekananda, Raja Yoga is the best of them. He considered it a "practical and scientific" method for which "no faith or belief is necessary."[9] "Rāja-Yoga," Vivekananda said, "is the only science of religion that can be demonstrated; and only what I myself have proved by experience, do I teach."[10]

Maintaining Neo-Vedanta's underpinnings of science, rationalism, and individualism, which it inherited from its English-educated founders, Vivekananda described yoga as a scientifically based system of spiritual growth. He offered yoga as a series of techniques each person could experiment with for themselves and then objectively verify its results.

Vivekananda talked about the role of the energy body and the kundalini in enlightenment, but, as his guru had taught him, he wasted little breath or ink on Hatha Yoga. At this time, the most visible Hatha yogins were the street yogis, performing their tricks and outrageous contortions for money. Vivekananda saw Hatha Yoga as serving very little purpose in the pursuit of spiritual liberation. [11]

Who He Taught

The Parliament of Religions was a two-week-long series of lectures by representatives of different faiths. It was held during the day, and this little fact turned out to be pivotal. Holding the lectures during the day meant that a considerable portion of the audience was made up of middle- and upper-class women, because at this point in history they were unlikely to have day jobs. And these ladies loved Vivekananda. They hung on his every word. The organizers quickly learned to schedule him at the end of the day so that the women would stay through the other speakers.

At this time in the northeastern U.S., there were several new psychospiritual movements afoot; Christian Science, New Thought, Spiritualism, and Mesmerism were all really popular, especially with middle- and upper-class women. And these were the people who took Vivekananda under wing, gave him room and board, created a buzz about him, and arranged speaking engagements for him. From the beginning of yoga in America, women have been at its heart.

Because of his proximity to these *fin de siècle* spiritual movements, Vivekananda necessarily defined his teachings as similar to or different from them. He went so far as to adopt the language and possibly even practices of some to help him relate to his audience and eventually his closer students. For example, tenets of New Thought, such as positive thinking, setting clear intentions, and using affirmations found a happy home in American yoga.[12]

Vivekananda wrote four books, one for each type of yoga, and he established Vedanta centers on both coasts. Even though he spent fewer than six years in the West, his formative influence on our current understanding of yoga is unmatched. And when he returned to India he was greeted as a hero and a saint—the swami who took Hinduism to America. His version of yoga, spliced as it was now with American popular spiritual psychology, took root in yoga's home country. It was Vivekananda's work and writing that initiated the yoga renaissance.[13]

Swami Vivekananda returned to India in 1900. America would have to wait decades for another emissary from India. While World War I put a damper on the East–West flow of people and ideas, the severe immigration restrictions of the National Origin Act and the Asian Exclusion Act of the early 1920s crushed it entirely.

Looking Ahead

And so we watch yoga continue to adapt and grow. Born as a mental discipline, it adapted to devotionalism and the Karma Yoga of the *Gita*. It reached out from the philosophies of Patanjali and Shankara to the tantric embrace of the world it once tried to escape. And then it came back, to the intense solitary strivings of the Hatha yogins. In this chapter we have watched it go from the yogin's hut, to the warrior ascetics of the Mughal Empire, to the street yogi of the British Raj. It's gone from Unitarian academics, to Neo-Vedanta translators, to heady Transcendentalists, to the front rooms of New England doyennes, and back again to middle-class, English-speaking India. And it never left any of its metamorphoses behind, but brought them all along—containing and offering all of these different paths toward communion with the Sacred.

We are now at the turn of the 20th century. Over the next fifty years, covered in the next two chapters, we will watch as yoga keeps adapting to new conditions, continuing to make its way from the Himalayas to Hollywood and from caves to community centers.

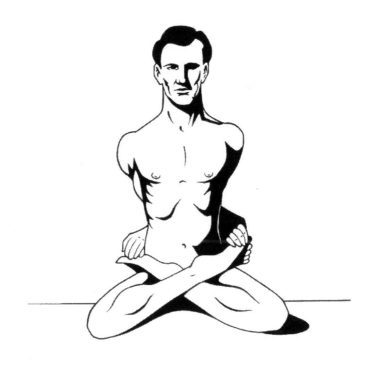

Theos Bernard in Baddha Padmasana

9 WESTERN SEEKERS, EASTERN LIGHTS

Welcome to the 20th century! Because of the whacked-out immigration laws in the first half of the 1900s, it makes sense to divide the story for this time period into two parts: (1) yoga from a Western perspective and (2) the changes that were going on in India. In this chapter we'll look into the former and next chapter the latter.

We will begin with the story of Hindu missionary Paramahansa Yogananda, who is most well-known for his book *Autobiography of a Yogi*. Then we visit Pierre Bernard, the first Hatha Yoga teacher in the U.S. We follow this up by looking into the yoga training Pierre's nephew, Theos Bernard, received in India. And finally we hear from a dialogue between a British reporter / spiritual seeker and an Indian hatha yogi. My intention in presenting these snapshots is to give us an idea of what yoga looked like to Americans in the first half of the 20th century.

Paramahansa Yogananda

Just like Vivekananda, Paramahansa Yogananda came to the U.S. to speak at a conference. His goal was to spread the teachings of yoga in the West. Before Neo-Vedanta, there were no Hindu missionaries, and since Yogananda, none have been as successful. Paramahansa is an honorific title that means "Great Swan." It signifies the highest level of spiritual realization and was given to Yogananda by his guru Sri Yukteswar.

In 1920, twenty-six years before the publication of his *Autobiography of a Yogi*, Yogananda arrived in Boston as a delegate to the International Congress of Religious Liberals. He stayed on in America, going on the lecture circuit and founding the Self-Realization Fellowship (SRF). Yogananda's teachings blended Neo-Vedanta, the tantric ideas of the energy body and kundalini, elements of Christianity, and astrology.

Let's spend a moment on these last two. Yogananda believed all authentic religions and scriptures pointed toward the same truth. He was especially taken with the story of Jesus, who he saw as a realized God-man. He published a two-volume commentary on the New Testament, and all of his works are peppered with quotations and stories from the Bible.

As for astrology, what is being referred to here is *jyotisha* (jyotiṣa), which is Hindu or Vedic astrology. It is different from Western astrology in a few important ways. It's based on the position of constellations rather than the sun and planets; a person is identified by their ascendant sign rather than their sun sign; and it is more interested in predicting large-scale future events in a person's life than psychological characteristics. (The marraige of yoga and Western astrology that is present in some branches of modern American yoga became prevalent in the 1970s through yoga's linking with the New Age movement.)

Throughout this amalgamation of ideas, Yogananda's focus remained on the inner divinity that all people share.

Kriya Yoga

Yogananda claimed Kriya Yoga as his lineage. The fundamental ideas of this Kriya Yoga differ substantially from that of Patanjali. In fact, they are the same as those of Neo-Vedanta:

~ God is the Absolute and the substance of all creation.
~ Each of us has a soul that is God within.
~ Spiritual development should be approached scientifically, by which he meant experimentally, so each person can discover what works best for them.
~ All religions are true.

Also new with this formulation of Kriya Yoga is the idea that certain kriyas or techniques can significantly speed up progress along the path of spiritual development, as we see in this passage of his *Autobiography*:

The *Kriya Yogi* mentally directs his life energy to revolve, upward and downward, around the six spinal centers (medullary, cervical, dorsal, lumbar, sacral, and coccygeal plexuses) which correspond to the twelve astral signs of the zodiac, the symbolic Cosmic Man. One-half minute of revolution of energy around the sensitive spinal cord of man effects subtle progress in his evolution; that half-minute of *Kriya* equals one year of natural spiritual unfoldment.[1]

Perhaps in part due to the growing American inclination toward immediate gratification, and doubtlessly because of his compassionate and authentic nature, Yogananda connected with tens of thousands of souls hungry for spiritual progress. Soon, the SRF had physical locations on both coasts and, new for its time, a correspondence / mail-order arm allowing it to reach people throughout the country and the world. The SRF also eventually established monastic facilities in California.

Yogananda, like Vivekananda, didn't have much to say about Hatha Yoga. He did believe people need to be in good physical shape to support their spiritual practice and toward this end developed what he called the Yogoda System, which was a combination of relaxation, breathing, stretching, strengthening, and concentration exercises.[2] But he steered clear of the larger system of Hatha Yoga, not seeing it as serving much purpose toward spiritual development.[3]

Still, he is strongly connected to modern postural yoga in America. His brother, Bishnu Ghosh, was a bodybuilder turned yoga teacher and taught none other than the notorious Bikram Choudhury, whom we'll talk about in the chapter on American yoga. And at least two students in Yogananda's lineage, J. Donald Walters and Melvin Higgins (who both went by the name Kriya-nanda), started organizations outside of the SRF that promoted asana along with the other methods Yoga-nanda taught.

Paramahansa Yogananda continued on in the U.S. for the rest of his life. Since his passing in 1952, the SRF has expanded to over five hundred temples and centers around the world. The mail-order lessons are still available through the SRF website. His many books are still available. *Autobiography of a Yogi* has been contin-uously in print for more than sixty-five years in multiple versions and languages. More than four million copies have been sold, and it's now in the public domain and available free online. It remains an important door to yoga for seekers around the world.

Now, switching gears from the saintly to the showman, we turn to the first American Hatha Yoga teacher—the Omnipotent Oom!

Pierre Bernard

The year is 1889 and the setting is the Midwest—Lincoln, Nebraska to be exact. It is here that we meet the 13-year-old boy, Perry Baker, who would become Pierre Arnold Bernard. Young Perry was fascinated by all things occult, and in a striking instance of the teacher appearing when the student is ready, a Syrian-Indian tantric Hindu by the name of Sylvias Hamati lived across the street from the Baker family. How Hamati came to be living in Lincoln is lost to history. Perry quickly became Hamati's devoted student, and in 1893, when Baker was 17, the two began traveling together. Perry Baker became Pierre Arnold Bernard, and the U.S. was about to see the first of many morally ambiguous homegrown gurus.

In 1907, after eighteen years with Bernard, Hamati returned to India. Bernard carried Hamati's picture with him his whole life.

Sensationalism and Scandal

Pierre Bernard first splashed across newspaper headlines in 1898 following a demonstration of his truly stupendous yogic powers. In front of an audience of doctors in San Francisco, he used pranayama to slow his heart rate so it could no longer be found. At that point, one of the doctors proceeded to sew through Bernard's upper lip. Experiencing no pain and little bleeding, Bernard made quite an impression.

He used the publicity from this exploit to begin a tantric lodge where he taught yoga. (This was the heyday of lodges and secret societies like the Freemasons and the Golden Dawn.) But it wasn't long before Bernard was faced with scandal and had to leave town.

Here we go! Right off the bat, American yoga is associated with sensationalism and accusations of sexual misconduct. Bernard and his followers were also run out of Seattle, Tacoma, and Portland because scandal, or at least rumor of scandal, followed them everywhere. Either because Bernard never dissuaded anyone from calling him "Doctor," a title to which he had no claim; or because he sent his more handsome male students to recruit young, preferably wealthy females; or because word got out that Tantra advocated ritualized sex—for any or all of these reasons, Bernard and his people were chased out of town after town.

So he did what any American would do if they wanted the freedom to practice something weird and taboo—he went to New York City. Even in this metropolis, though, Bernard was accused of immorality. This time it was because he had apparently promised to marry two different young women, and they found out about each other. They had him charged with abduction and sent to prison. At least that's one version of the story.

Pierre Bernard, derisively nicknamed the Omnipotent Oom by the press, was imprisoned for months until the charges were finally dropped, but the damage to his name and to the popular opinion of yoga was done.

Bernard Finds His Home

Slowly, Bernard rebuilt his reputation enough to start a school for yoga and Sanskrit. He trained female dancers as yoga instructors and gave lectures himself on philosophy. A large portion of his clientele was upper-class women.

In 1918 Bernard opened what would come to be called the Clarkstown Country Club, with financial help from his wealthier patrons, including the Vanderbilts. The CCC, as members called it, was situated in Nyack, New York, about an hour's drive north of New York City. It was part ashram for spiritual seekers and part sanitarium for wealthy socialites suffering from depression or "nerves," a.k.a. anxiety. P.A., as Pierre was now called by club members, married Blanche de Vries, a one-time follies dancer, and under their charge the country club thrived.

The Teachings

Bernard's teachings were tantric through and through. He believed, as Hamati had taught him, that the goal of life is to realize that the world is sacred and the place to start is within.

In fact, as we heard in chapter 7, according to his biographer Robert Love, Bernard believed "the material world is lit to its atoms by the spark of God. The key to the mystery of life—if you care to know it—is this unrealized unity. Our tragedy is that we fall for the illusion of separateness—*maya* in Sanskrit."[4]

To foster this realization of unity, the students at the CCC studied Sanskrit texts and practiced asana, pranayama, and meditation. They also worked hard and played hard, holding circuses, theatrical performances, grand galas, and baseball games.

Bernard held lectures in his study that went far into the night. And he and de Vries continued to train the next generation of yoga teachers (most with dance backgrounds) and send them out to NYC, the Midwest, and as far as California to teach others. The asana they taught were those from the classic texts.

Upshot

Pierre Bernard was a character, a plain Midwesterner

who told people he was God and so are you. He pros-
pered through the Depression and saw his dreams
realized in the material realm, at least for a while. He
used good old American showmanship, drive, and self-
assuredness to get the ball rolling on the business of
yoga in America.

Bernard was also a publicity hound and, at least in
his early years, a hound dog. But his dedication to yoga
never failed. He was a good student for his guru and a
willing teacher, especially if you had money. But
because of Bernard we can say that, from the very
beginning, yoga in America has been permeated by
scandal, shady publicity stunts, and marketing based on
current standards of beauty. American yoga seems to
have always had this strange mix of sincerity and
narcissism.

Theos Bernard

Pierre Bernard had a brother, Glen, who was also a
dedicated yogi. Glen was involved in the initial days of
the tantric lodges, but he left Pierre to his shenanigans
early on. Glen held firmly to the belief that yoga is a
secret and solitary undertaking. It never sat right with
him that Pierre had monetized the teachings.

In 1908, Glen had a son whom he named Theos
Casimir Bernard. I'll refer to him as Theos or Theos
Bernard to avoid confusion with his uncle Pierre. Best
known for his exploits as the "White Lama," Theos con-
tributed significantly to the academic field of Tibetan
studies. But before all that, he trained in India in the

traditional style of Hatha Yoga and wrote about his experience for his doctoral dissertation at Columbia University. It's a fascinating read that provides a window into Hatha Yoga just before its total renovation.

We'll switch gears now, hunkering down into the fine details of Theos Bernard's experiences in India in 1936–37, with an eye toward gaining an appreciation of just how much the process of learning yoga has changed over fewer than a hundred years.

On Retreat

In his published thesis, *Hatha Yoga: The report of a personal experience*, Theos Bernard tells us he undertook his "retreat," as he calls it, in Ranchi. After being introduced to his potential teacher, whom he calls simply Maharishi, he was interviewed at length. The guru took Theos on as a student only after being convinced of his preparation in and commitment to yoga.

Before entering the more advanced training, Theos had some work to do. For three weeks he followed a preparatory schedule. First, he had to master the shat karma of purification. During these initial days, he would wake at 4:00 a.m. and do the cleansing practices of dhauti, neti, and basti. Then he would perform uddiyana bandha and nauli, followed by viparitakirani (head stand) for half an hour. This session would end with 10 rounds of bhastrika (bellows breath) at 100 breaths per minute and retention of the breath for a minute each round.

After this Theos would study until 10:30 a.m., when he would again perform head stand for 30 minutes, 10 rounds of bhastrika, and then asana. Following this, he would rest, have lunch, and read until 4:00 p.m., when he would once again practice uddiyana bandha and nauli; another 30 minute head stand, which he eventually increased to an hour at each go; and 10 more rounds of bhastrika, increasing gradually to 120 breaths per minute for three continuous minutes followed by breath retention for five minutes.

Still in this preliminary stage, he was instructed to do a variation of trataka to establish himself in concentration. Here is his description of the "candle exercise":

In preparation for practicing contemplation, my teacher recommended what is commonly known as the "candle exercise," which I was to use every evening before retiring. It is a simple technique for establishing an afterimage on the retina, which you are supposed to watch with fixed attention until it disappears. Place a lighted candle some eighteen inches in front of you on a level with your eyes and stare at the flame until tears begin to flow. Then close your eyes with cupped hands and watch the mental image. The problem is to try to hold the image still. It is permissible to move it backward and forward, but it must not be allowed to move sideways or up and down.[5]

After three weeks of preparation, he started the advanced series of exercises.

Asana

In his first month of retreat, the emphasis was on physical training. He doesn't give a schedule of his days during this time, except to say he added a midnight session to his program.

Theos was given asana to practice that he describes as falling into three categories. First he was instructed in postures meant "to bring a rich supply of blood to the brain and to various parts of the spinal cord."[6] These were:

- ~ Sarvangasana (sarvāñgāsana): shoulder stand
- ~ Halasana (halāsana): plow pose
- ~ Paschimottanasana: intense stretch of the west posture or posterior stretch
- ~ Mayurasana: peacock pose

Then he learned the "reconditioning" postures, which were meant "to stretch, bend and twist the spinal cord in different ways." These were mostly prone back-bends, except the last:

- ~ Shalabhasana: locust pose
- ~ Bhujangasana: cobra pose
- ~ Dhanurasana: bow pose
- ~ Ardha matsyendrasana: half Lord of the Fishes pose or half-spinal twist

For these two sets of postures, both of which focus on the spine, he explains his approach as follows:

I tried to hold each posture ten seconds and then repeated the practice five times. This was enough in the beginning. Later I increased the time until I could hold each position comfortably for one minute, repeating them ten times without fatigue. After I developed sufficient strength to hold sarvāṅgāsana, I raised the time to fifteen minutes instead of repeating it several times, as I did with all the other āsanas.[7]

When Theos demonstrated the necessary mastery of these asana, he moved on to the meditation postures, of which there were only two: siddhasana and padmasana. About the latter he says:

Many months were required for the perfection of this posture. By "perfection" I mean the state of accomplishment given by Vyāsa [in his commentary on the *Yoga Sutras*], "posture becomes perfect when effort to that end ceases, so that there may be no more movement of the body." The requirement that the posture must be held for three hours is the chief difficulty and makes intelligible why it took so long to achieve it.[8]

It quickly becomes clear that asana used to be held much longer than they are in modern postural yoga classes. After demonstrating sufficient mastery of padmasana, Theos was assigned the following:

~ Kukkutasana: cock pose
~ Uttanakurmakasana: raised tortoise pose
~ Yogasana: cross-legged forward fold, sometimes called yoga mudra
~ Vajroli mudra: which looks like a variation of boat pose
~ Pashini (pāśini) mudra: noose mudra, these days often called yoga nidrasana

Theos notes that head stand, which he also practiced, is not classified as an asana but as a mudra and that, as with padmasana, the "standard for perfection is three hours," which he eventually worked up to.

Pranayama and Mudras

Besides asana, Theos was taught several types of pranayama and mudras. The first breathing exercise was alternate nostril breathing, which was presented as a preparatory, cleansing practice to be done before pranayama. The following is a list of the breathing exercises he learned; the translations are those he uses. All of these come straight from the classic Hatha Yoga texts.

~ Surya bhedana: piercing the solar disc
~ Ujjayi: victorious
~ Sitkari: hissing
~ Shitali: cooling
~ Bhastrika: bellows
~ Bhramari: bee
~ Murchha: faint

The mudras he was assigned were as follows:

~ Mahamudra
~ Mahabandha
~ Mahavedha, which is assuming mahabandha in padmasana and using the hands on the floor to lift the seat a few inches and let it drop back to the floor repeatedly. This could more easily be called butt bouncing. The aim is to jar the kundalini loose.
~ Khecari mudra, which he managed by lengthening his tongue, cutting the frenum a little bit every day with a razor blade until he could curl it back into the esophageal passage.
~ Viparitakarani
~ Shaktichalani (śakticālani), which is performed in baddha (bound) padmasana, with the arms wrapped around the back and hands grabbing the toes of the feet from behind, right hand to right toes and left to left. (See this chapter's illustration.) All of the bandhas are then engaged. The yogi spends an hour and a half in this position working directly with the kundalini.

And I Still Haven't Found . . .

Theos was young and strong. He was completely committed to the practice and followed his guru's instructions to the letter. But Theos Bernard was looking for magic. He wanted to find the siddhis, the supernatural abilities yogis are famous for, and to his vast disappointment, he didn't experience any. His retreat with the Maharishi lasted only three months, and while he'd practiced quite a bit beforehand and continued to afterward, he gained only radiant physical health and clarity and calmness of mind. His teacher explained that it could take many years of devoted work to gain what Theos Bernard was looking for.

While he never stopped being a yogi, Theos returned to life in America, hopped on the lecture circuit, and finished graduate school. When he finally did return to India in 1947, he went missing in newly created Pakistan and was never heard from again.

A Search in Secret India

Taking with us what we've gathered about Hatha Yoga as practiced in ashrams in the early 20th century from Theos Bernard's account, we turn to another. This one, which is from the perspective of an Indian yogi, comes from Paul Brunton's 1935 book, *A Search in Secret India*. Brunton was a British journalist and a spiritual seeker. He is credited with bringing the great sage Ramana Maharshi and his meditation method of continuously asking "Who am I?" to the attention of the Western world.

Brunton devotes nearly thirty pages to his interviews with a hatha yogi named Bramasuganandah, whom he calls simply Brama. Brama, Brunton tells us, is physically fit and reticent to speak. He looks to be in his mid-30s but is really nearer to 50. Brunton has to rely on a translator, which may explain the yogi's sometimes stilted speech. Another note on translation: Brunton calls

Hatha Yoga "the Yoga of Body Control."

As they begin their conversation, Brama is at pains to make Brunton understand that whatever he thinks he knows about Hatha Yoga, it probably isn't the real deal. Brama says:

The Yoga of Body Control is little understood except by the adepts who have mastered it, and the common people possess the most false notions of our ancient science. And since adepts are, alas! so infrequently to be found to-day, the most foolish and distorted practices pass as our system without hindrance among the multitude. Go to Benares and you will see a man who sits all day and sleeps all night on a bed of sharp spikes; and in another place you will see a man who holds one arm aloft in the air until it is half withered from disuse and until the nails are several inches long. You will be told that they are men who practice our system of Yoga, but it is not so. Such men bring shame on it, rather. Our aim is not to torture the body in foolish ways for the sake of public wonder; these self-torturing ascetics are ignorant men who have picked up by hearsay, or from some friendly person, a few exercises in the forced contortion of the body. But since they know not what are our objects, they distort these practices and prolong them unnaturally. Yet the common people venerate such fools and bestow food and money on them.[9]

When Brunton presses him for details about his beliefs and practices, Brama responds,

> Ours is the most secret of all the Yogas; it is full of grave dangers, not only to the disciple himself, but to others. Think you that I am allowed to reveal any but its most elementary doctrines to you, or even those without extreme discretion?

What he can share, he says, are the beginning practices meant to strengthen the will and the physical body:

> We have four kinds of exercises or methods to accomplish this early work of putting the body's health in good order. First we learn the art of repose so that the nerves may be soothed. . . . Then we learn the "stretches," which are exercises copied from the natural stretching of healthy animals. Third we clean the body thoroughly by a variety of methods which may seem very curious to you, but which are indeed excellent in their effect. Lastly, we study the art of breathing and its control.[10]

In other words, relaxation, asana, shat karma, and pranayama.

Brama goes on to explain that the first step is to adopt a posture that is completely relaxed and free of strain. He describes three postures appropriate to relaxation: sitting cross-legged, sitting with the knees pulled up under the chin and ankles crossed, and shavasana. Then, he says, you must "withdraw your thoughts from all worldly burdens and affairs; just rest your mind on a beautiful object, a picture or a flower."[11]

"By practice," he says, "you may learn to rest in any of these attitudes for an hour, if you wish. They take away tension of muscle and soothe nerves. Repose of muscle comes before repose of mind."

Brunton protests, "Really, your exercises seem to consist of nothing more than sitting still in some way or other!"

"Is that nothing?" Brama responds. "You Westerners thirst to be active, but is repose to be despised? Do calm nerves possess no meaning? Repose is the beginning of all Yoga, but it is not our need alone; it is also the need of your world."

Brunton concedes that he's got a point. [12]

The Purposes of Postures

Brama tells Brunton that there are eighty-four asana, of which he knows sixty-four. Unfortunately, we are not privy to the names of these postures. When asked the purpose of the postures, Brama responds that they are useful for awakening "deep power," which probably means the kundalini, and also for removing impurities and maintaining or restoring health:

The mere fact of sitting or standing for regular periods in certain fixed postures may seem of small importance in your eyes. But the concentration of attention and will power upon the chosen posture is so intense—if success is to be gained—that sleeping forces awaken within the Yogi. Those forces belong to the secret realms of Nature, therefore they are seldom fully aroused until our breathing exercises are also practised, for the breath possesses deep powers. Though the awakening of such forces is our real aim, no less than a score of our exercises are capable of being used for benefiting one's health or to remove certain diseases; while others will drive impurities out of the body. Is this not of great use? Still other postures are intended to assist our efforts to get control over the mind and soul, for it is a truth that the body influences thought no less than thought influences the body. In the advanced stages of Yoga, when we may be plunged for hours in meditation, the proper posture of the body not only enables the mind to remain undistracted in its efforts, but actually assists its purpose. Add to all these things the tremendous gain in will power which comes to the man who perseveres in these difficult exercises, and you may see what virtues there are in our methods.[13]

Asana versus Physical Culture

To understand the next part of their discussion, we need to introduce the concept of "**physical culture**." Physical culture was a Western health and strength-building movement that included calisthenics, gymnastics, and weightlifting among other exercise systems. In the early decades of the 20th century, physical culture was all the rage in Britain and the U.S., as well as a few continental European locations including Scandinavia and Germany. It played an enormous role in the development of modern postural yoga, and we'll talk more about it in just a few pages. But for now we know enough to understand what he meant when Brunton asked Brama what the difference was between yoga asana and this British way of exercising.

Our Yoga exercises are really poses and require no further movements after the pose has been taken up. Instead of seeking more energy with which to be active, we seek to increase the power of endurance. You see, we believe that though the development of the muscles may be useful, it is the power which is behind them that is of greater value. Thus if I tell you that standing on your shoulders in a particular way will wash the brain with blood, soothe the nerves and remove certain weaknesses, you as a Westerner would probably do the exercise for a moment and repeat it several times with a rush. You may strengthen the muscles which are called into action by this exercise, but you would get little of the benefits which a Yogi gets by doing it in his own way.[14]

"And what may that be?" Brunton asked.

"He will do it slowly, with deliberation, and then maintain this position as steadily as he can for some minutes." Brama goes on, "The difference between the two ways is shown by the soothing effect of the posture upon the brain and nerves."

Finally, when, on the last day of their interviews, Brunton presses Brama to reveal his "deeper secrets,"

Brama asks, "Are you ready to abandon the life of cities and to retire into a solitary place in the hills or the jungle for some years?"

When Brunton hesitates, Brama continues, "Are you ready to give up all other activities, all your work, renounce your pleasures and put your whole time into the exercises of our system—and that not merely for a few months, but for several years?"

"I do not think so," Brunton says. "No—I am not ready. One day, perhaps——"

"Then I can take you no farther. This Yoga of Body Control is too serious to become the mere sport of a man's leisure hours."[15]

Same Time, Different Place

Is it irony that in the next chapter we turn to the beginning of the movement that made Hatha Yoga a class at the Y?

Because of the dearth of information flowing from India to the U.S., in the first half of the 20th century huge developments were afoot in the realm of Hatha Yoga of which we had very little knowledge. Plus, not many would have cared. But while occasional truth seekers from the West were heading East to find enlightenment, freedom seekers of India were turning to Hatha Yoga to gain the strength to win their independence.

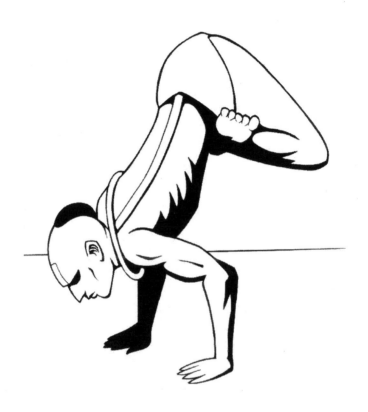

Krishnamacharya in Vrscikasana

10 THE BIRTH OF MODERN POSTURAL YOGA

Yoga has always been a dynamic tradition, growing and changing to meet people's needs. In early 20th century India, yoga was used to serve needs very different from those of its past. Instead of spiritual liberation, yoga was recruited to serve as a tool for political liberation.

In the late 1800s and early 1900s, the Indian Independence Movement was growing. The British in India had perpetuated a stereotype of the Indian people as weak and submissive. With the physical culture movement prompting the English to get fit "for God and country," this supposed physical weakness was seen as a moral failing and a sign that India needed, if not deserved, the strong ruling hand of the British. The outlook behind the physical culture movement was so pervasive that the English-educated nationalist Indians took for granted that to win independence, they needed to build the physical strength of their populace.[1]

Let's recall here that the physical culture movement was a health and strength training campaign in the U.S., England, and a few continental European countries. Various physical disciplines were created or updated to get the middle and upper classes, whose lives had become increasingly sedentary, moving and fit. Weight lifting, calisthenics, gymnastics, stretching, and breathing exercises as well as fencing, boxing, and wrestling were promoted through both private gymnasiums and the YMCA, which was founded in the mid-1800s. Physical culture also included such influential ideas as muscular Christianity and the nature cure movement, which were just what they sound like.

Leaders of the Indian Independence Movement didn't have to look far for an indigenous equivalent to the British fitness regimens. Hatha Yoga presented the perfect solution—a native system that was imbued with the spiritual culture of Hinduism. By this point the exercises of Hatha Yoga had already been used by groups of warrior ascetics and may have already been cross-pollinated with elements of the indigenous Indian wrestling system. For sure it picked up the *danda* (daṇḍa) exercises from the latter, which is where the seeds of the modern *surya namaskara* come from. As Mark Singleton tells us in his intriguing and rigorous investigation into this time frame:

The creator of the modern *sūryanamaskār* system, Pratinidhi Pant, the Rajah of Aundh, was himself . . . a devoted bodybuilder and practitioner of the Sandow method [weight lifting], and he went on to definitively popularize the dynamic sequences of *āsana* that have become a staple of many postural yoga classes today.

He goes on, making the point abundantly clear:

Sūryanamaskār, today fully naturalized in inter-national yoga milieu as a presumed "traditional" technique of Indian yoga, was first conceived by a bodybuilder and then popularized by other body-builders, . . . as a technique of bodybuilding.[2]

Through the work of several freedom-seeking edu-cators, asana practice became amenable to the average person by drawing from traditional Hatha Yoga texts, European gymnastics, and Indian wrestling.[3] A further development of this time, due to widespread English-language education in India, is that English became the common language of yoga. Again, this was the case so that Indians who spoke different languages and dialects could communicate with each other. It was just a side effect that it made modern postural yoga available to the entire English-speaking world.

There are four figures through whom we can trace the transition into modern postural yoga: Shri Yogendra, Swami Kuvalayananda, Sivananda Saraswati, and Tiru-malai Krishnamacharya. The first two changed how yoga is thought about and practiced in India, and the students of the second two would extend yoga's reach around the world.

Medicalization of Asana

Shri Yogendra and Swami Kuvalayananda characterize the effort to harness yoga toward the goals of Indian independence and make it relevant to the public at large. As medical anthropologist Joseph Alter points out, it was in India that yoga was modernized, medicalized, and transformed into a system of physical culture.[4]

At the turn of the last century, yogis were considered social pariahs, littering cities with the spectacle of their unsightly contortions and severe deformities caused by extreme austerities. And the Hatha Yoga texts promise magical powers and immortality, things quite at odds with early 20th century scientific rationalism. In order for Hatha Yoga to play a part in the revolution, it needed a makeover. And while men like Yogendra and Kuvalayananda very purposefully shifted the focus away from street yogis and magic and toward yoga's promise of radiant health, they never intended to remove or even overlook its spiritual core.

Shri Yogendra

Shri Yogendra founded the field of yoga therapy. As a student, he was an athlete and a skeptic. His skepticism subsided when he met his guru, Sriman Parmahamsa Madhavdasji Maharaj, known better as Madhavdasji. Madhavdasji had been a civil servant before taking sannyasa and spending years practicing yoga while wandering the Himalayas. Yogendra never took sannyasa but worked for Madhavdasji in a clerical capacity. He eventually married and had children, which led in no small way to his contribution of adapting yoga to the life of householders.

In 1918, Yogendra opened the Yoga Institute in Santa Cruz, a neighborhood of Bombay (now Mumbai), where he taught asana classes in a physical education format, free to anyone and everyone. He also trained teachers at the Institute and began using asana and pranayama as tools for physical therapy.

In 1920, Yogendra traveled to New York, where he opened another Yoga Institute just thirty miles from Pierre Bernard's thriving Clarkstown Country Club. Also in common with Bernard, to secure funding for the center he used the impressive physical abilities he had gained from his own practice to demonstrate the power of yoga. According to Alter,

> [A] number of leading physicians were invited to the flat where he was staying on Riverside Drive to watch as he inflated one lung at a time, changed the temperature of extremities at will, turned on lights with the electricity from his body, and stopped his watch.[5]

The display must have been convincing because support was quickly forthcoming.

The Yoga Institute in Harriman, New York, was, like Bernard's CCC, part ashram and part sanitarium. During the three years he ran the center, Yogendra (called Yogananda at the time) worked closely with an American doctor, an experience that greatly expanded his knowledge of the therapeutic possibilities of yoga.

233

He also came into contact with all of those turn-of-the-century psychospiritual movements, like Spiritualism, Mesmerism, and New Thought, that Vivekananda had encountered, and found himself defining yoga as similar to or different from them.

After New York, Yogendra returned to the Yoga Institute in Santa Cruz, where he continued to teach, research, and write about the healing benefits of yoga. After living his entire life as a householder holy man, he passed on in 1989, and the Yoga Institute continues on today, as strong and relevant as ever.

Swami Kuvalayananda

Swami Kuvalayananda is significant for beginning laboratory research on yoga. He founded Kaivalya-dhama Health and Yoga Research Center in 1924. As a student, Kuvalayananda had been strongly attracted to the nationalist movement as well as to the cause of physical fitness in the name of winning independence. As a young man he took a vow of celibacy and committed to the following three goals:

(1) Prepare the young generation for service of the country; (2) master the Indian system of physical education and integrate it with general education; and (3) bring together science and spirituality by coordinating the spiritual aspects of Yoga with modern science.[6]

Already well on his way to participating in the yoga renaissance, he met Madhavdasji, who became his guru also. As a byproduct of his intense practice, Madhavdasji had developed siddhis and suggested to Kuvalayananda that he should study these supernatural side effects of yoga scientifically.

And that is how Kaivalyadhama came to serve at least four different purposes in the propagation of yoga: as a center for teaching yoga as physical fitness; a training center for the mass production of yoga teachers; a laboratory for documenting the therapeutic benefits of asana, pranayama, and dhyana; and the first research center to study the parapsychological effects of yoga.

Shortly after opening Kaivalyadhama, Kuvalayananda moved away from identifying his work with the nationalist effort and reimagined his vision as serving all of humankind. Kuvalayananda passed on in 1966, and Kaivalyadhama remains an important institution to this day.

While Yogendra and Kuvalayananda changed the face of yoga in India, our next two subjects, Swami Sivananda Saraswati and Tirumalai Krishnamacharya, both established lineages that would go on to propagate this new form of yoga in America and worldwide.

Swami Sivananda Saraswati

The boy who would become Swami Sivananda Saraswati was born in 1887. He was raised and educated in southern India. As a kid, he excelled in academics and gymnastics. At university he studied medicine, and he went on to be a physician in Singapore, which was at that time part of British Malaya. After ten years he resigned and went to Rishikesh, where he took sannyasa and devoted himself to his own and others' spiritual liberation.

Sivananda never did stop being a doctor, though, and often used his knowledge to help those in need, especially fellow mendicants. His background as a physician also informed his belief that physical health is fundamental to the spiritual quest.

It didn't take long for Sivananda to attract a following. Rishikesh is an important pilgrimage site; however, not all of the travelers who recognized Sivananda as their guru could pack up and move there. Between the need to communicate with these people and his deep desire to persuade Indian youth to adhere to traditional Hinduism, Sivananda started to write. At first he wrote pamphlets but quickly escalated to books. He wrote with astonishing speed. By the time he passed on, Sivananda had written over three hundred books in English.[7]

He wrote a book about everything we have talked about in this book and more. One of his early works was called *Yogic Home Exercises: Easy course of physical culture for men and women*.[8] Sivananda expounded on history, morality, and dharma. He translated and wrote commentaries on the Upanishads, the *Ramayana*, the *Mahabharata*, the *Bhagavad Gita*, the *Yoga Sutras*, the Tantras, and more. He saw all of it as fitting into one whole, one gestalt, of Hindu spirituality. But the *Yoga Sutras* and Vedanta had the greatest impact on the religious philosophy he lived and taught.[9]

The more he wrote, the more popular he became. Sivananda was sought out by seekers the world over, including Mircea Eliade, who was a formative figure in the field of Religious Studies and the author of *Yoga: Immortality and freedom.* As more and more people continued to gather around him, it became necessary for Sivananda to set up some kind of organizing structure. That is how he came to found the Divine Life Society (DLS) in 1936, an organization that continues today and has branches all over the world.

The Teachings

Sivananda advocated an all-encompassing approach to spiritual life. Here is one summary of Sivananda's instructions:

> [T]o get up before sunrise, do *yogasana*, specially the *Padmasana*, *japa*, and meditation; observe dietary rules, *brahmacharya*, *ahimsa*; keep fast and silence; study and learn the Hindu sacred texts and scriptures; and live a life of simplicity, sacrifice and of surrender to God.[10]

In this way, Sivananda brought together several of the various threads of Hinduism and yoga. But his most important contribution may have been his emphasis on ahimsa, which he translated as love and saw as the most powerful force in the world. In his own words:

> Ahimsa is Supreme love. Ahimsa is Soul-force. Ahimsa is divine life. Hate melts in the presence of love. Hate dissolves in the presence of Ahimsa. There is no power greater than Ahimsa. The practice

of Ahimsa develops will-power to a considerable degree. The practice of Ahimsa will make you fearless. He who practices Ahimsa with real faith can move the whole world, can tame the wild animals, can win the hearts of all, can subdue his enemies. He can do and undo things. The power of Ahimsa is ineffable. Its glory is indescribable. Its greatness is inscrutable. The force of Ahimsa is infinitely more wonderful and subtle than electricity or magnetism.[11]

After millennia of gurus and texts emphasizing detachment, Sivananda's emphasis on ahimsa and love might have been exactly what the occupants of the Kali Yuga needed to hear. While Sivananda was a sannyasin who practiced renunciation, celibacy, and complete dedication to the spiritual life, he taught householders as well. The Divine Life is open to all.

Sivananda's Lineage

Many of Sivananda's disciples would go on to create their own organizations and styles of yoga. Swami Sivananda Radha founded the Yasodhara Ashram in Canada. She also published several books including *Hatha Yoga: The Hidden Language*. Swami Vishnu-devananda developed Sivananda Yoga, and Swami Satchidananda started Integral Yoga, both of which are alive and well in the U.S. today.

The schools of yoga that descend from Sivananda's lineage are characterized by their inclusion of yogic philosophy and ethics. Their practices include deep relaxation, mudras, chanting, meditation, and diet as well as asana and pranayama. Asana practice favors function over form, and as students progress, poses are held for longer durations. Some include a form of surya namaskara.

Tirumalai Krishnamacharya

T. Krishnamacharya was born the year after Sivananda, in 1888. One predominant theme of his young life was education. His first guru was his father, a teacher of the Vedas. With his father, little Krishnamacharya studied Sanskrit and the sacred texts, and learned asana and pranayama. His father passed on when Krishnamacharya was only ten.

Krishnamacharya went on to study all six schools of Hindu philosophy and became a master of *Ayurveda,* the indigenous Indian medical system. As a young man, he spent seven and a half years living with his guru and the guru's family in a Himalayan cave, where he studied the *Yoga Sutras*, practiced asana and pranayama, and learned the therapeutic uses of yoga. When he left, his teacher instructed him to marry, have children, and teach yoga. So that is what he did.

At first, there was no work to be found as a yoga teacher, and Krishnamacharya earned money for his family as a foreman on a coffee plantation. On his days off he gave lectures and exhibitions. According to writer Fernando Pagés Ruiz:

These demonstrations, designed to stimulate interest in a dying tradition, included suspending his pulse, stopping cars with his bare hands, performing difficult asanas, and lifting heavy objects with his teeth. To teach people about yoga, Krishnamacharya felt, he first had to get their attention.[12]

Eventually Krishnamacharya came under the patronage of the Maharaja of Mysore, who hired him to teach asana to the boys at the palace school and to popularize yoga around India by giving exhibitions. Before long, Krishnamacharya was given his own *yogashala* (yogaṣala), or place for yoga. It is here that he began refining postures, experimenting with sequencing, and combining pranayama and asana.

He also began adopting and adapting techniques to meet his students' needs. The palace had a long tradition of supporting indigenous arts and an extensive library of books on both native and nonnative systems of physical culture. There were also other styles of physical education, such as wrestling, on offer in close proximity to Krishnamacharya's classes.

Krishnamacharya's overarching theme was healing. It was his intention to meet students where they were and give them what they needed to be as healthy as possible. He saw every person as unique and thought the role of a good teacher was to identify how yoga can best help them achieve optimal well-being. Krishnamacharya's lineage is best described through four of his students who went on to popularize yoga across the globe: Krishna (K.) Pattabhi Jois, Bellur Krishnamachar

Sundararaja (B. K. S.) Iyengar, Indra Devi, and Tiru-
malai Krishnamacharya Vendata (T. K. V.) Desikachar.

K. Pattabhi Jois

Hired to teach yoga to school-age boys, Krishnamacharya adapted surya namaskara into the aerobic, athletic
practice of vinyasa. Vinyasa is characterized by flowing
movements between asana that are coordinated with the
breath. It incorporates many strong standing and balance
postures that Krishnamacharya adopted from European
gymnastics and other systems of physical culture.

One of the boys Krishnamacharya taught was K.
Pattabhi Jois. Jois learned the primary, intermediate, and
advanced series of vinyasas and, beginning in 1937,
went from being one of the boys to teaching the boys.
Jois claimed to have never deviated from the sequences
he learned from Krishnamacharya. He named his style
Ashtanga Yoga (sometimes Ashtanga Vinyasa), which
points to the significance that both Krishnamacharya and
Pattabhi Jois gave to the eight limbs of yoga from
Patanjali's *Yoga Sutras*. Jois' Ashtanga Yoga became
increasingly popular in the U.S. in the last quarter of the
20th century, finding adherents in gym culture, as we'll
see in the next chapter, as well as in celebrities like Sting
and Madonna.

B. K. S. Iyengar

Also during this early period of Krishnamacharya's
teaching, while he was still at the yogashala in Mysore,
his young, sickly brother-in-law came to stay with him.
B. K. S. Iyengar proved to be proficient at asana, and

Krishnamacharya used to take him on what he called his "propaganda tours." Iyengar wasn't with Krishmacharya very long before he returned to full health, and soon after that he became a teacher. Even though he was only 18 in 1937 when he was sent far away from Mysore to Pune to teach on his own, the young Iyengar must have been at least a little relieved to be out from under the famously terse and demanding Krishnamacharya.[13]

Iyengar developed his own style of asana class, dropping vinyasas in favor of focusing on alignment. In 1952 his student and friend, violinist Yehudi Menuhin, brought Iyengar with him to Switzerland, which turned out to be a pivotal moment leading to opportunities to teach throughout Europe and the U.S. Then, in 1966, Iyengar's bestseller *Light on Yoga* was published, solidifying his predominant role in the worldwide spread of yoga in the 20th century.

Indra Devi

In 1938, the year after Pattabhi Jois and Iyengar starting teaching, and at the direct request of the Maharaja, Krishnamacharya took on his first female student, who also happened to be his first Westerner. Russian-born Eugenie Peterson, who would become Indra Devi, studied with Krishnamacharya for a year. When she learned her husband was being relocated to China, Krishnamacharya told her she should start teaching. She spent several days with Krishnamacharya, hurriedly writing as he dictated everything he felt she needed to know.[14]

Devi learned a gentler kind of yoga from Krishna-macharya than what he taught the school boys. The instruction he gave her was based mostly on the asana from the traditional Hatha Yoga texts. So that is what she taught, in China and then in Hollywood.

First Pierre Bernard trained young, female dancers to be yoga teachers, and then Devi became the "First Lady of Yoga" by teaching movie stars like Eva Gabor and Greta Garbo. And this is how modern yoga ended up being introduced to the American public at large through the idealized feminine body.

T. K. V. Desikachar

Krishnamacharya had six children. The one who would do the most to facilitate and perpetuate his father's work was T. K. V. Desikachar. Desikachar was born in 1938, the same year Devi became a student. At this point, Krishnamacharya was continuing on under the good graces of the Maharaja. That changed after Independence in 1947, when he lost funding for his books and his yogashala. Making his way by taking on individual clients, Krishnamacharya solidified his reputation as a healer.

In his youth, Desikachar was not interested in yoga. It was only around 1961, after finishing a degree in engineering, that he witnessed the healing and joy his father's work created in others and decided to study with him. According to Desikachar, Krishnamacharya had mellowed quite a bit as he was forced out of the shala and into the homes of individual clients. Desikachar studied and trained with Krishnamacharya for thirty years, longer than anyone else. At this point in his teaching, Krishnamacharya was a master at meeting people where they were, adapting the yoga to their limitations, and challenging them back to health.

Desikachar would go on to found the Krishnamacharya Yoga Mandiram Institute of Yoga and Yoga Studies to continue his father's work and lineage.

Wait, What Just Happened?

Something major shifted with the adaptation of Hatha Yoga into the realm of physical culture and the Indian Independence Movement. Hatha Yoga was no longer secret but had become publicly available. Like with the ascetic mercenaries, it was not a solitary practice but done in groups. It was no longer necessary to renounce the world; no longer necessary to make a lifelong commitment; no longer necessary to be accepted by a guru and receive initiation. All a student of Hatha Yoga had to do was show up to class.

The teachers were different too. While Yogendra, Kuvalayananda, and the other teachers we met in this chapter dedicated their lives to the practice, study, and teaching of yoga, they never claimed enlightenment. And while they deeply believed they were offering the whole package of Hatha Yoga in a form accessible to householders, they were also redefining it in a way that shifted the focus more and more toward the physical practice and its benefits.

Whereas the texts of Hatha Yoga make it clear that the physical practices come prior to and are subservient to the mental disciplines, what comes out of the Hatha Yoga renaissance of the early 20th century is, to borrow Alter's phrasing, "metaphysical fitness and physical philosophy." As much as no one meant for it to happen, we've started down the road that will lead, in many situations, to the whole of the practice getting crammed onto the mat. By the mid-20th century, the sprawling, magical, powerful liberation tradition that was Hatha Yoga is well on its way to being compacted into the format of a P.E. class.

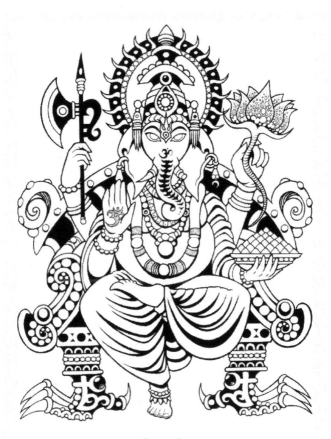

Ganesha

11 AMERICAN YOGA

All right dear readers, we're nearing the present. Over the second half of the 20th century, yoga went from being an obscure Eastern concept to a household word and everyday practice for millions of Americans. In this chapter we'll look at the major elements of American yoga decade by decade. We'll see that, through the '50s, '60s, and '70s, yoga followed the counterculture. Metaphorically speaking, it could be said that, if yoga did drugs, in the '60s he was that weird guy in the corner who we were all pretty sure was stoned. Then he joined the New Age movement and tripped balls. In the '80s, yoga got caught up in the mainstream, took cocaine, went to the gym, and got sweaty. And in the '90s, and even probably up until today, yoga is still trying to get clean and rescue his soul from the capitalist marketplace.

We begin in mid-century . . .

1950s

Pierre Bernard, Indra Devi, and a few others had tried to bring the benefits of yoga to the attention of the American public. And to a small extent they had succeeded. For the interested demographic, information about yoga and other Eastern philosophies was becoming more available. It also started to take hold in the arts and avant-garde.

Paramahansa Yogananda's *Autobiography of a Yogi* came out in 1946, and Aldous Huxley, who was deeply influenced by yoga, wrote about the bigger spiritual picture in *The Perennial Philosophy* (1945) and *The Doors of Perception* (1954). Alan Watts published with *The Way of Zen* in 1957. The '50s was the decade of the Beat poets, who discovered Eastern philosophy through the Transcendentalists and ran with it. Jack Kerouac's *Dharma Bums* came out in 1958.

On the asana front, Walt and Magaña Baptiste, who had started the first gym to incorporate yoga in 1934, opened the first yoga school in San Francisco in 1955. Walt had been Mr. Universe in 1949 and was well known in the world of physical culture. The Baptistes continued the connection between asana and physical fitness that began in India at the turn of the century. Their three children all went on to become acclaimed yoga teachers.

1960s

In the '60s, yoga blossomed along with the flower children. As the Maharishi Mahesh Yogi became famous as the guru to the Beatles and the Beach Boys, yoga was introduced to a whole new generation of Americans, a generation that would look to the East for answers to both ultimate questions like the meaning of life and political questions like racism and war. The Maharishi developed Transcendental Meditation (TM), which thrived in the '60s and '70s and eventually became a multibillion-dollar business. The TM organization spawned several important names in the self-help world, like John Gray of *Men Are from Mars, Women Are from Venus* fame and Deepak Chopra, famous for being Deepak Chopra.[1]

It was also in the '60s that Amrit Desai founded the Kripalu Center for Yoga and Health, named after his guru, Swami Kripalvananda. The Kripalu style of yoga was developed specifically for Westerners. It's a slow, mindful style that has three stages, culminating in the practice of asana as spontaneous meditation in motion. Desai left the community in 1994 after a sex-related scandal. Management of the center was taken over by students and teachers, and Kripalu continues to be a strong and well-respected organization and school.

The '60s saw the publication of Iyengar's *Light on Yoga*, with descriptions of two hundred asana, which is still the standard for many today. Iyengar also started traveling to facilitate teacher trainings in the '60s. On one such occasion in London, he was asked to avoid talking about religion or spirituality. He agreed. Later he explained, "Better life can be taught without using religious words. Meditation is of two types, active and passive. I took the active side of meditation by making students totally absorbed in the poses."[2] This might have been a pivotal moment in both how classes are taught and how teachers are trained, unintentionally shifting the focus away from personal transformation and toward perfecting the postures.

On the other side of the coin, the Sikh master Yogi Bhajan, founder of Kundalini Yoga, emigrated to Canada in 1968 and established the Healthy, Happy, Holy Organization (3HO) in 1969. Kundalini Yoga is an overtly spiritual practice, which attempts to awaken the kundalini through dynamic kriyas that include asana, pranayama, mantra, and meditation. The goal is to experience God in this lifetime. During Yogi Bhajan's lifetime, more than a hundred 3HO ashrams were established in North America with another two hundred spread around the world.

In 1969, Swami Satchidananda, founder of Integral Yoga and a carrier of the Sivananda Saraswati lineage, opened Woodstock. Mainstream American culture might not have been ready for yoga, but the seeds were planted and the generation of love was primed to bring yoga with it as they moved kicking and toking into adulthood.

1970s

Ram Dass née Richard Alpert's story is an iconic representation of the yoga experience in the early 1970s. Originally a professor at Harvard, in the late '60s, Alpert was in on the beginning of LSD experimentation with Timothy Leary. Looking for natural rather than drug-induced enlightenment, he went to India where he found his guru in Neem Karoli Baba and became Ram Dass. His classic *Be Here Now* was published in 1971. Since then Ram Dass has spent his entire life advocating and facilitating spiritual awakening.

During the '70s yoga became suffused throughout the New Age movement, which is itself an extension of those same movements, such as Spiritualism, Mesmerism, and especially New Thought, that Vivekananda and other early harbingers encountered and defined yoga in relation to. Western astrology, crystals, the rainbow color scheme of the chakras—all this and more was grafted onto yoga in the '70s.

Outside of the counterculture, the '70s also saw the introduction of yoga into the American home through Richard Hittleman's *Yoga for Health* television series and Lilias Folan's long-running PBS show, *Lilias, Yoga and You*. Yoga on TV made it accessible and more acceptable to middle- and upper-class housewives across the nation.

And finally, Bikram Choudhury got his start in the '70s. Choudhury was a student of Bishnu Ghosh, Paramahansa Yogananda's brother. Choudhury, known for founding Bikram Yoga, might have been the first person to set out to purposefully develop a brand of yoga. In Bikram Yoga, a series of 26 postures is performed in a room heated to 105° Fahrenheit. Bikram Yoga became steadily more popular through the '80s and '90s. Eventually, Choudhury tried to copyright his posture sequence but lost his case in 2015. At the time of this writing, Choudhury is being sued by several former students and employees under allegations of sexual harassment, assault, and rape.[3]

1980s

In the '80s, yoga in some ways continued to expand and in others continued to contract. Beryl Bender Birch, a student of Pattabhi Jois, popularized Power Yoga, and Baron Baptiste, son of Walt and Magaña, trademarked Baptiste Power Vinyasa Yoga. Power Yoga is athletic and aerobic, so it was an easy fit into the surge of gym culture across the country. However, what went into the gyms was a narrow version of asana practice, often trimmed of nearly all spiritual content. But true to form, yoga never discarded the old while adopting the new, and teachers of the slower styles of asana continued to offer classes out of their homes and studios.

It was in this decade that Hatha Yoga became a description for classes that weren't Power or Vinyasa or Bikram or otherwise branded, which has caused its fair share of confusion as newcomers try to figure out how all of these different practices relate to each other. Also during the '80s, specialized types of practices started to gain ground, such as prenatal yoga, kids yoga, yoga for runners, yoga for back care, and so on. Creating forms of yoga that are accessible and beneficial to various populations is a current that has only grown stronger with time.

1990s

In the '90s, the yoga boom picked up momentum. The

increase in teacher trainings prompted the organization of the International Association of Yoga Therapists (1989) and Yoga Alliance (1999). The scent of profits led to yoga-themed clothing and lifestyle brands like Lululemon and Gaiam and to training franchises like YogaFit and YogaWorks.

Typifying the decade was the uber-popular Anusara brand. Created by John Friend and drawing especially from the Krishnamacharya-based schools, Anusara incorporates vinyasa and alignment as well as ideas about spirituality and community garnered from tantric sources. Anusara was attractive because once again yoga was bringing together body and soul. It continued to gain in popularity through the '90s and led the way in Internet-based classes. Friend, however, was accused of sexual and financial misconduct and stepped down from his position in 2012.[4] Even though the organization is now in the hands of its constituents, many Anusara-trained teachers have distanced themselves from the name.

The New Millennium

Now, here we are. This is where our history stops, because it's the present. Everything from here on isn't history but commentary, observations without the assistance of a window of time through which to gain perspective. However, without going too far out on a limb, it can be said that yoga in America has both issues and potential, and will probably have both for the foreseeable future.

Issues

American yoga has issues: body issues, guru issues, money issues, cultural appropriation issues, just a whole lot of issues. And this is in no small way because yoga—once secret and sacred—is a business in the U.S. The yoga industry is swollen with books (like this one), magazines, clothing lines, gear brands, and retreat get-aways, to say nothing of the proliferation of teacher trainings. Companies seek out the strongest, most flexible bodies with the serenest faces to be their "brand ambassadors." And in the process they've created the phenomenon of rock star yogis and further perpetuated the image of the yoga practitioner as conforming to or even surpassing mainstream standards of beauty.

And it doesn't stop there. Yoga is used not just to sell more yoga, but to sell anything and everything. The transition is complete. The naked sannyasin alone in the forest seeking ultimate freedom in union with the Sacred has transmogrified into a skinny white woman with a bare midriff in a glossy ad for high-end kitchen appliances, or a luxury car, or a computer.

And in rebuttal, there is a well-intentioned movement to make yoga accessible to everyone equally, regardless of their physical appearance or abilities. But some of these efforts have gone so far in their attempts to make yoga not just accessible but palatable to all comers that they have further stripped the physical practice of any spiritual content.

According to one perspective, it's enough to just do the poses mindfully. But if that were the case, wouldn't gymnasts be experiencing spontaneous kundalini awakenings?

As we've seen throughout the history of yoga philosophy, intention matters. The desire to be free of suffering and willing to work for it are early steps on the path. Morality and stillness, nurturing detachment and compassion, and fostering the experience of samadhi— these have been present in all the various manifestations of yoga throughout history.

Where is the study or devotion or even action? If it isn't Jnana or Bhakti or Karma, if it isn't Tantra, breaking down societal constructs and embracing the whole of creation as sacred, is it yoga?

Has yoga lost its way? Have we lost something fundamental to yoga? And if so, when did the devolution begin? Was it when the ascetic warriors co-opted the physical disciplines of Hatha Yoga to their struggles? Was it when the Neo-Vedantists democratized Jnana Yoga, making it equally available to all? Was it when the leaders of the yoga renaissance adapted asana to the cause of independence? When Pierre Bernard and Indra Devi attached the practice to the bodies of dancers and starlets? When the Baptistes opened the first gym that offered yoga classes? When Iyengar agreed to leave the spiritual content out of his teacher training in London? Was it Power Yoga? Bikram Choudhury? Lululemon's ultra-sheer hundred-dollar yoga pants?

Potential

Yoga is a dynamic tradition. It adapts to the needs of the people who practice it. Throughout its history, yoga has subsumed new disciplines while never getting rid of old ones. As long as it keeps leading people to quieter minds and along the spiritual path, it keeps being yoga.

Even if the majority of Americans who come to yoga begin for the health benefits or the desire for a lithe "yoga body," many hang around for the deeper effects. In a time when stress is epidemic and our entire financial system is based on marketers making us feel insufficient, some are drawn to yoga as an escape out of their heads and into their bodies. For some it is healing and comforting. And there will always be those who start to dig deeper and find this vast, compelling history. They will find the gods and goddesses and engage in the rigors of study and the discipline of contemplation. They will undertake the process of emptying of self to let the Sacred shine through. And maybe some will go even further, to the ultimate goal of all yoga—liberation.

AFTERWORD

There you have it, the story of yoga in broad strokes and bright colors. And just like every story based on history, this is a snapshot of what we know at this moment. Work continues, though. Archeologists, cultural anthropologists, linguists, and historians will continue to fill in and modify the picture. Dates for texts will most likely change. Old theories will be set aside so new, hopefully more accurate ones can take their place. And the story will continue to evolve as it moves into the future.

So take this as a best guess, from one limited perspective, of how yoga originated, grew, and spread around the world.

And still it is my fervent hope that you, dear reader, have walked through the door this book provides, into a room full of other doors; that you will pick up and delve deeply into the Upanishads, the *Gita*, the *Yoga Sutras*, and the classic texts of Hatha Yoga; and that you will continue to open the doors of yoga, both outside and in.

END NOTES

Introduction

1. Years given are a simplified version of those in Feuerstein, *Study Guide for The Yoga Tradition*. The only major alteration I made was changing Feuerstein's Sectarian Age (1300 – 1700) to the Empiric Age (1300 – 1800) because our focus narrows around developments pertaining to Hatha Yoga at this point, and the political reality of empires has more influence on the story than the religious phenomenon of sectarianism.

2. BCE stands for Before Common Era. It replaces BC and is an attempt to refer to dates as currently understood without blatantly deferring to any religion in the process. CE means Common Era and replaces AD to refer to dates this side of Jesus.

3. The term "modern postural yoga" comes from Elizabeth de Michelis.

4. Feuerstein, *The Yoga Tradition*, 91.

5. Tilak Pyle, *The Online Sanskrit Pronunciation Guide*, 2007, http://tilakpyle.com/sanskrit.htm.

6. Olivelle, *Katha Upanishad*, p. 246, chap. 6, verse 11.

Chapter One

1. Eliade, *Shamanism*.

2. Feuerstein, Kak, and Frawley, *In Search of the Cradle of Civilization*.

3. Panikkar, *Rig-Veda*, 10.129, in *The Vedic Experience, Mantramañjarī*, p. 58.

4. Ibid., 10.90, p. 75.

5. Ibid., 1.164, p. 660.

6. Ibid., 10.136, pp. 436-37.

Chapter Two

1. Radhakrishnan and Moore, "Laws of Manu," 177-84.
2. Olivelle, *Brihadaranyaka Upaniṣad,* 1.4.10, p. 15; 2.5.19, p. 33; and 2.5.14, p. 32.
3. Easwaran, *Chandogya Upanishad,* 6, pp. 131-39.
4. Easwaran, *Brihadaranyaka Upanishad,* 4.4, pp. 114-15.
5. Feuerstein, *The Yoga Tradition,* 69.
6. Easwaran, *Brihadaranyaka Upanishad,* 4.4.5, p. 114.
7. Olivelle, *Taittirīya Upanishad,* 1.9, p. 182.
8. Easwaran, *Chandogya Upanishad,* 1.1.1, p. 125.
9. Olivelle, *Brihadaranyaka Upanishad,* 6.8.2, p. 152.
10. Olivelle, *Kauṣītaki Upaniṣad,* 2.1, p. 206.
11. Ibid., 2.5, p. 208.
12. Easwaran, *Chandogya Upanishad,* 7.26.2, p. 141.
13. Olivelle, *Taittirīya Upanishad,* 2.7-8, pp. 188-89.
14. Easwaran, *Taittirīya Upanishad,* 2.4.1, p. 253.
15. Olivelle, *Brihadaranyaka Upanishad,* 4.5.6, p. 70; 4.5.15, p. 71.
16. Easwaran, *Brihadaranyaka Upanishad,* 4.3.21-22, 4.3.32, 4.4.23 4.4.5, pp. 111-15.

Chapter Three

1. Menon, "Kishkinda Kanda," in *The Ramayana.*
2. Menon, "Uttara Kanda," in ibid.
3. Easwaran, *The Bhagavad Gita,* 3:27-28, p. 107.
4. Ibid., 6:23-25, p. 142.
5. Ibid., 16:1-4, p. 238.
6. Ibid., 16:21-22, p. 241.
7. Ibid., 3:25, p. 107.
8. Ibid., 3:19, p. 106.
9. Ibid., 2:49-50, pp. 94-95.
10. Ibid., 18:47-48, p. 262.

11. Ibid., 9:27-28, pp. 176-77.
12. Ibid., 4:11, p. 117.
13. Ibid., 6:28-29, p. 143.
14. Ibid., 2:52-64, pp. 95-96.
15. Ibid., 5:25-26, p. 130.
16. Ibid., 8:22-23, p. 168.
17. Ibid., 8:9-10, p. 166.

Chapter Four

1. Feuerstein, Sutra 1.2, *The Yoga Tradition,* 217.
2. Hartranft, *The Yoga-Sūtra of Patañjali*, 2.
3. Prasad, "The Yoga Sūtra," 454.
4. Feuerstein, *The Yoga Tradition*, 222.
5. Radin, *Supernormal*, 113.
6. Feuerstein, *The Yoga Tradition*, 254.
7. Ibid., 224.
8. Feuerstein, *The Encyclopedia of Yoga and Tantra*, s.v. "Tapas," 371.
9. Sutra 2.46.
10. Feuerstein, *The Yoga Tradition*, 313-16.
11. Hartranft, Sutra 2:49.

Chapter Five

1. Feuerstein, *The Yoga Tradition*, 171.
2. Prabhavananda and Isherwood, *Shankara's Crest-jewel of Discrimination*, 44.
3. Ibid, 94.
4. Ibid, 51.
5. Ibid, 93.
6. Ibid.
7. Ibid, 91.

Chapter Six

1. Avalon, *The Great Liberation,* 11.
2. Feuerstein, *The Encyclopedia of Yoga and Tantra,* s.v. "Kali-Yuga," 178.
3. Ibid., s.v. "World ages," 411.
4. Woodroffe, *Introduction to Tantra Śāstra,* 5.
5. Woodroffe, *Tantrarāja Tantra,* xv.
6. Feuerstein, *The Encyclopedia of Yoga and Tantra,* s.v. "Panca-ma-kāra," 256-57.
7. Avalon, *The Serpent Power,* 317-488.
8. Ibid., 355.
9. Ibid., 317-488.
10. Feuerstein, *The Yoga Tradition,* 360.
11. Woodroffe, *Introduction to Tantra Śāstra,* 126.
12. Love, *The Great Oom,* 162.

Chapter Seven

1. Prabhavananda and Isherwood, *Shankara's Crest-jewel of Discrimination,* 45.
2. Ibid., 102.
3. Feuerstein, *The Yoga Tradition,* 384.
4. Ibid., 382-83.
5. Vasu and anon., *Siva Samhita,* 30.
6. Ibid., 31.
7. Csikszentmihalyi, *Flow.*
8. Vasu, *Gheranda Samhita,* 46.
9. Svatmarama, *Hatha Yoga Pradipika,* 81.
10. Ibid., 83.
11. Vasu, *Gheranda Samhita,* 49.
12. Ibid.
13. Svatmarama, *Hatha Yoga Pradipika,* 90.
14. Ibid.

15. Vasu, *Gheranda Samhita*, 50.
16. Svatmarama, *Hatha Yoga Pradipika*, 181.
17. Mallinson, *Gheranda Samhita*.
18. Svatmarama, *Hatha Yoga Pradipika*, 196.
19. Ibid., 201.
20. It is likely that this passage is an interpolation of the translator.
21. Svatmarama, *Hatha Yoga Pradipika*, 78-81.
22. Ibid., 21.

Chapter Eight

1. Singleton, "Fakirs, Yogins, Europeans," in *Yoga Body*.
2. Pennington, *Was Hinduism Invented?*
3. Mather, "India Christiana."
4. Walton, "Unitarianism and Early American Interest in Hinduism."
5. Emerson, "Brahma."
6. Thoreau, *Walden,* 312.
7. Syman, *The Subtle Body,* 33.
8. Walton, "Unitarianism and Early American Interest in Hinduism."
9. Vivekananda, "Raja-Yoga," in *The Complete Works of Swami Vivekananda.*
10. Vivekananda, "Inspired Talks," in ibid.
11. Syman, *The Subtle Body,* 74.
12. De Michelis, *A History of Modern Yoga,* 116.
13. Ibid., 182.

Chapter Nine

1. Yogananda, *Autobiography of a Yogi,* 267.
2. Yogananda, *Yogoda or Tissue-Will System of Physical Perfection.*

3. Syman, *The Subtle Body,* 171.
4. Love, *The Great Oom.* 162.
5. Bernard, *Hatha Yoga,* 54-55.
6. Ibid., 7.
7. Ibid., 8.
8. Ibid., 10.
9. Brunton, *Search in Secret India,* 75.
10. Ibid., 76.
11. Ibid., 77.
12. Ibid., 78.
13. Ibid., 80.
14. Ibid., 81.
15. Ibid., 99.

Chapter Ten

1. Brunton, *Search in Secret India,* 82-83.
2. Singleton, *Yoga Body.*
3. Sjoman, *The Yoga Tradition of the Mysore Palace,* 60.
4. Alter, *Yoga in Modern India,* 10.
5. Alter, "Shri Yogendra."
6. Alter, *Yoga in Modern India,* 82.
7. Gyan, *Sivananda and His Ashram,* 12.
8. Sivananda, *Yogic Home Exercises.*
9. Gyan, *Sivananda and His Ashram,* 13, 69.
10. Ibid., 135.
11. Ibid., 55.
12. Ruiz, "Krishnamacharya's Legacy."
13. Iyengar, *Light on Life*, xix.
14. Ruiz, "Krishnamacharya's Legacy."

Chapter Eleven

1. Goldberg, P. *American Veda.* 174.

2. Newcombe, "The Institutionalization of the Yoga Tradition."
3. Ceasar, "Yoga Guru Bikram Choudhury Must Pay $6.4 Million in Punitive Damages, Jury Decides."
4. Roig-Franzia, Manuel, "Scandal Contorts Future of John Friend, Anusara Yoga."

GLOSSARY

Abhyasa (abhyāsa): spiritual practice

Advaita: "not two," nondual, relating to the metaphysical position that there is only one substance, **Brahman**

Ahimsa (ahimsā): "nonharming," the first **yama** in the eight limbs of Patanjali's *Yoga Sutras*

Ajna: "command," the sixth **chakra**, which is located at the level of the forehead

Anahata: "unstruck (sound)," the fourth **chakra**, which is located at the level of the heart

Anatman (anātman): "no self," the Buddhist idea that there is no soul

Anubhava: direct experience; according to Vedanta, a direct experience of the knowledge that atman and Brahman are identical

Aparigraha: "greedlessness," one of the **yama** in the eight limbs of Patanjali's *Yoga Sutras*

Asamprajnata (asanprajnāta): "without content," refers to the unitive state **samadhi** without cognitive content in *Yoga Sutras*

Asana (āsana): "posture," meditation posture

Ascetic: self-discipline and abstention from indulgence, a person who practices such

Ashtanga: "eight limbs," refers to the eight limbs of yoga in Patanjali's *Yoga Sutras*

Asteya: "nonstealing," one of the **yama** in the eight limbs of Patanjali's *Yoga Sutras*

Atman (ātman): the individual soul; the true Self

Avatar: an earthly incarnation of a deity

Avidya: "no knowledge," ignorance

Bandha: energy locks made by contracting certain parts of the body

Bhakta: one who practices **Bhakti Yoga**

Bhakti Yoga: the path of divine love, characterized by qualified nondual or dualistic **metaphysics** and the practices of worship, prayer, and contemplation of the divine form

Bhoga: enjoyment, refers to the idea in Tantra Yoga that spiritual life should include both bhoga and yoga, enjoyment and discipline

Brahmacharya (brahmacarya): celibacy, chastity,

Brahman: the Sacred, the Absolute, the ground of existence, God

Brahmin: a priest of the Vedic religion, belonging to the priestly **caste**

Caste: hereditary classes of Hindu society

Chakra: energy center in the **subtle body** along the spinal axis

Darshana: "view," used to refer to any of the six philosophical schools of Hinduism or to seeing a deity or holy person

Deva: deity, masculine form

Devi: deity, female form

Dharana: concentration as a spiritual practice

Dharma: duty, virtue upholding cosmic order

Dhyana (dhyāna): the state of absorption in meditation

Dualism: the metaphysical position that two separate types of substances exist, e.g., mind and matter, God and creation

Esoteric: understood only by those with special knowledge

Gunas: the three qualities of nature, the actions of which are responsible for everything in the created, material world

Hatha Yoga: the yoga of force, characterized by a nondual **metaphysics** and the use of physical practices such as the **shat karma** and **asana** as preparation for higher mental practices

Hinduism: the many religious and cultural traditions of the Indian subcontinent that trace their lineage back through the *Bhagavad Gita*, the Upanishads, and the Vedas

Ida: one of the **nadis** that spirals up the spinal axis, originating on the left side of the body, where prana flows along with the **pingala** when the **sushumna** is blocked by the **kundalini**

Ishta devata (iṣṭadevatā): "cherished deity," an individual's chosen deity

Ishvara (Īśvara): "Lord," a special instance of **Purusha** in the *Yoga Sutras*

Ishvara pranidhana (Īśvara pranidhāna): devotion to the Lord, one of the **niyama** in the eight limbs of Patanjali's *Yoga Sutras*

Jalandhara (jālandhara) bandha: throat lock or chin lock, contracting the throat by pulling the chin inward

Japa: repetition, the practice of repeating a **mantra**

Jivan mukti (jīvan mukti): living liberation, the idea that individuals can attain **moksha** while still in human form

Jnana (jñāna): knowledge, wisdom

Jnana Yoga: the path of knowledge, characterized by a nondual philosophy and the practices of renunciation, study, and meditation

Jyotisha (jyotiṣa)**:** Hindu or Vedic astrology, differs from Western astrology in being based on stars instead of planets and more interested in long-range events than personality characteristics

Kaivalya: aloneness, liberation from **samsara** in the *Yoga Sutras*

Kali Yuga: according to Hindu cosmology, the current degenerate world age, the final of the cycle of four

Kama: love, desire

Karma: action, the effects or consequences of our actions

Karma Yoga: the path of self-transcending action

Keshins: long-haired **ascetics** referred to in the Vedas, possible forerunners of yoga

Kirtan: a call-and-response style of yogic chanting

Klesha: "afflictions," causes of suffering according to the *Yoga Sutras*

Kriya: action toward spiritual progress, refers to the metaphysics and practices of Patanjali's *Yoga Sutras* as well we to the branch of yoga brought to the U.S. by Paramahamsa Yogananda

Kshatriya: the warrior class of the Hindu **caste** system

Kumbhaka: breath retention

Kundalini (kuṇḍalini)**:** "serpent," "coiled one," the form of **Shakti** that lays dormant at the base of the **sushumna** which the practices of **Tantra** and **Hatha Yoga** seek to awaken

Loka samgraha: "world gathering," promoting the welfare of the world

Mahabandha: "great lock," performing all three **bandhas** simultaneously

Mahasiddhis: "great powers," usually refers to supernatural powers

Mahasiddhas: a person who has attained moksha and developed supernatural powers

Mahavakyas: "great sayings," verses from the Upanishads used as objects of meditation in **Vedanta**

Mandala: symbolic diagram used in visualization

Manipura: "city of jewels," the third **chakra**, which is located at the navel or solar plexus

Mantra: sacred sound or word, used in **japa** and **kirtan** spiritual practices

Math: monastery

Maya: appearance, illusion, signifies the unreality of the created world

Metaphysics: the study of what is, of the substance of what exists

Moksha (mokṣa)**:** spiritual liberation

Mudra: energy seal, gesture used to control the flow of **prana**

Mukhya: "chief," refers to the early or primary Upanishads

Mula (mūla) **bandha:** root lock, contracting the anal sphincter and lifting the pelvic floor

Muladhara: "root support," the first **chakra**, which is located at the perineum

Nadis: channels through which **prana** flows in the **subtle body**

Neo-Vedanta: the reformulation of **Vedanta** from the mid-1800s that places individual experience as primary

Nirguna: "without qualities," used by Shankara to describe the formless nature of **Brahman**

Nirvana: "blown out," the Buddhist term for liberation from **samsara**

Nirvikalpa: the state of union, **samadhi,** with no cognitive content

Niyama: moral observances, the second limb of **Ashtanga Yoga** as listed in Patanjali's *Yoga Sutras*

Nondualism: the metaphysical position that everything that exists is of the same substance

Om: sacred **mantra** symbolizing the Absolute, said to be the sound at the center of creation

Padas: "feet," chapters in the *Yoga Sutra*

Pancha kosha (panca kosha): the five sheaths of the **subtle body,** the first description of the subtle or energy body, from the *Taitteriya Upanishad*

Physical culture: Western health and strength-building movement from the turn of the 20th century, which strongly influenced the creation of modern postural yoga

Pingala: one of the **nadis** that spirals up the spinal axis, originating on the right side of the body, where prana flows along with the **ida** when the **sushumna** is blocked by the **kundalini**

Prakriti: the created world, mind and matter

Prana: life energy

Pranayama (prāṇāyāma): breathing exercises, the practice of controlling the breath

Pratyahara (pratyāhāra): sense-withdrawal, the practice of withdrawing attention from the senses and turning inward

Purusha: "Cosmic Man" in Vedas, another name for the Sacred Absolute thereafter

Qualified nondualism: the metaphysical position that while God and creation are of the same substance, God is more than creation

Rajas: active, excited, one of the **gunas** or qualities of nature

Rishi: sages who received the knowledge of the Vedas in ecstatic states, an honorific title for saintly yogins

Rita (ṛta): cosmic order

Sadhana (sādhana): an individual's particular spiritual practice or discipline

Saguna: "with qualities," used by Shankara to describe Brahman merged with **maya**

Sahasrara: "thousand petalled," the energy portal or seventh **chakra** located at or above the crown of the head

Samadhi (samādhi): the state of union, ecstasy, bliss

Samprajnata (samprajnāta): "with cognition," the state of union, **samadhi,** with cognition in *Yoga Sutras*

Samsara (saṁsāra): the ongoing cycle of birth, life, death, and rebirth

Samskara (saṃskāra): subliminal imprints or habits of mind

Samtosha: contentment, one of the **niyama** in the eight limbs of Patanjali's *Yoga Sutras*

Samyama: the process of meditation, its three parts are concentration, absorption, and **samadhi**

Sannyasin (saṁnyāsin): one who renounces social and material things to focus on spiritual liberation

Satchitananda: being, consciousness, bliss or truth, consciousness, bliss; refers to the state of union with Brahman

Sattva: lucidity, purity, one of the **gunas** or qualities of nature

Satya: truthfulness, one of the **yama** in the eight limbs of Patanjali's *Yoga Sutras*

Savikalpa: describes the state of union, **samadhi,** with cognitive content

Shakti (Śakti)**:** power, energy; the goddess who represents the feminine, creative aspect of the Sacred in **Tantra Yoga**

Shaman: gatekeeper to the spiritual realm in tribal societies

Shat karma (ṣaṭkarman)**:** "six actions," the six bodily purification practices of **Hatha Yoga**

Shaucha (shauca)**:** cleanliness, purity

Shiva (Śiva)**:** the god of destruction in the **trimurti,** Lord of Yoga, and the representation of the masculine and pure consciousness in **Tantra Yoga**

Shruti: "that which was heard," revealed texts

Shudra (śūdra)**:** servant class of the Hindu **caste** system

Siddha: perfected; a realized sage who has manifested **siddhis**

Siddhi: perfection, power, often a supernatural power

Smriti: "that which was remembered," texts that are considered to be written by human authors

Soma: drink with psychotropic qualities used in Vedic ceremonies, the deity of the intoxicating drink

Subtle body: the body belonging to each individual made of life energy or **prana**

Surya namaskara: sun salutation

Sushumna (suṣumṇa)**:** the central, spinal channel of the **subtle body**, through which the **kundalini** flows upon **samadhi** according to **Tantra** and **Hatha Yoga**

Sutra: "thread," a compact philosophical statement

Svadhistana: "own base" or "seat of the self," the second **chakra**, which is located at the level of the sacrum

Svadhyaya (svādhyāya): study; one of the **niyama** in the eight limbs according to Patanjali's *Yoga Sutras*

Tamas: lethargic, dark; one of the three **gunas** or qualities of nature

Tapas: heat, asceticism; the practice of spiritual discipline

Tantra: "loom" or "web," a sacred text in **Tantra Yoga**

Tantra Yoga: the radically nondual path, characterized by the belief that the material world / microcosm is equally sacred as the transcendent / macrocosm and by myriad practices including **mantra**, **mudra**, **yantras**, **mandalas**, and working with the **subtle body**

Tantrika: one who practices **Tantra Yoga**

Transcendentalism: an influential early American philosophical and literary movement that held idealism and individualism as central tenets, proponents of which were deeply influenced by early translations of yogic texts and influenced later Hindu popularizers

Trimurti: three forms, the three central deities of **Hinduism:** Brahma, Vishnu, and Shiva

Turiya: "the fourth," refers to the fourth state of consciousness, beyond waking, dreaming, and dreamless sleep; pure consciousness

Uddiyana (uddīyāna) **bandha:** stomach lock, pulling the abdomen in and up

Unitarianism: a radically monotheistic Christian denomination holding that each individual has a divine spark and should be free to follow the spiritual path to which they feel called

Untouchables: the class below the lowest **caste** of the Hindu social system

Vairagya (vairāgya): detachment or dispassion

Vaishya: the merchant class of the Hindu **caste** system

Varnas: castes of the Hindu social structure

Vedanta: "the end of the Vedas," one of the six philosophical schools of **Hinduism**, reiterates the worldview of the Upanishads

Vibhuti (vibhūti): psychic or paranormal power

Vidya: wisdom, knowledge

Vishuddha: "purity," the fifth chakra, which is located at the level of the throat

Vratyas (vrātyas): brotherhood of mystics written about in the Atharva Veda, possible forerunners of yoga

Yama: moral restrictions; one of the eight limbs in Patanjali's *Yoga Sutras*

Yantra: symbolic diagram used in visualization

Yoga: the mystical paths of spiritual traditions that began in India, the activity of seeking a direct experience of the Sacred

Yogi: a practitioner of yoga

Yogini (yogini): a female practitioner of yoga

Yuga: "age," one of the four divisions of the world cycle, according to Hindu cosmology

BIBLIOGRAPHY

Alter, Joseph S. "Shri Yogendra: Magic, Modernity, and the Burden of the Middle-Class Yoga." In *Gurus of Modern Yoga*, edited by Mark Singleton and Ellen Goldberg. Oxford: Oxford University Press, 2014. E-book.Alter, Joseph S. *Yoga in Modern India: The Body between Science and Philosophy*. Princeton, NJ: Princeton University Press, 2004.

Avalon, Arthur. *The Great Liberation (Mahānirvānā Tantra)*. 2nd ed. Madras: Ganesh & Co., 1927. First published 1913.

Avalon, Arthur. *The Serpent Power: The Secrets of Tantric and Shaktic Yoga.* 4th ed. Madras: Ganesh & Co., 1950. First published 1919.

Bernard, Theos. *Hatha Yoga: The Report of a Personal Experience.* New York: Columbia University Press, 1944.

Brunton, Paul. *Search in Secret India.* New York: E. P. Dutton & Co., 1943. First published 1935.

Ceasar, Stephen. "Yoga Guru Bikram Choudhury Must Pay $6.4 Million in Punitive Damages, Jury Decides." *Los Angeles Times,* January 26, 2016, http://www.latimes.com/local/lanow/la-me-ln-bikram-yoga-lawsuit-20160126-story.html (accessed May 6, 2016).

Csikszentmihalyi, Mihaly. *Flow: The Psychology of Optimal Experience.* New York: Harper & Row, 1990.

De Michelis, Elizabeth. *A History of Modern Yoga: Patañjali and Western Esotericism.* London: Continuum, 2004.

Desikachar, T. K. V. *The Heart of Yoga: Developing a Personal Practice.* Rochester, VT: Inner Traditions International, 1995.

Devi, Indra. *Forever Young Forever Healthy*. Englewood Cliffs, NJ: Prentice-Hall, 1953.

Dowman, Keith, trans. *Legends of the Mahasiddhas: Lives of the Tantric Masters*. Rochester, VT: Inner Traditions, 2014.

Easwaran, Eknath, trans. *The Bhagavad Gita*. 1st ed. Tomales, CA: Nilgiri Press, 2007.

Easwaran, Eknath, trans. *The Upanishads*. Tomales, CA: Nilgiri Press, 2007. First published 1987.

Eliade, Mircea. *Shamanism: Archaic Techniques of Ecstasy*. Princeton, NJ: Princeton University Press, 1964. E-book.

Eliade, Mircea. *Yoga: Immortality and Freedom*. New York: Pantheon Books, 1958. First published 1936.

Emerson, Ralph Waldo. "Brahma." http://www.poetryfoundation.org/poem/175138 (accessed April 27, 2016).

Feuerstein, Georg. *The Encyclopedia of Yoga and Tantra*. Boston: Shambhala, 2011.

Feuerstein, Georg. *Tantra: The Path of Ecstasy*. Boston: Shambhala, 1998.

Feuerstein, Georg. *The Yoga Tradition: Its History, Literature, Philosophy and Practice*. 3rd ed. Prescott, AZ: Hohm Press, 2008.

Feuerstein, Georg. *Yoga Morality: Ancient Teachings at a Time of Global Crisis*. Prescott, AZ: Hohm Press, 2007.

Feuerstein, Georg, Subhash Kak, and David Frawley. *In Search of the Cradle of Civilization: New Light on Ancient India*. Wheaton, IL: Quest Books, 1995.

Frawley, David. *Hymns from the Golden Age: Selected Hymns from the Rig Veda with Yogic Interpretation*. Delhi: Motilal Banarsidass, 1986.

Goldberg, Michelle. *The Goddess Pose: The Audacious Life of Indra Devi, Who Helped Bring Yoga to the West.* New York: Knopf, 2015.

Goldberg, Philip. *American Veda: From Emerson to the Beatles to Yoga and Meditation How Indian Spirituality Changed the West.* New York: Three Rivers Press, 2010.

Gyan, Satish Chandra. *Sivananda and His Ashram.* Madras: Diocesan Press, 1980.

Hartranft, Chip. *The Yoga-Sūtra of Patañjali: A New Translation with Commentary.* Boston: Shambhala, 2007.

Iyengar, B. K. S., with John Evans and Douglas Adams. *Light on Life: The Yoga Journey to Wholeness, Inner Peace, and Ultimate Freedom.* Emmaus, PA: Rodale Books, 2005.

Johnson, Willard. *Poetry and Speculation of the Rg Veda.* Berkeley, CA: University of California Press, 1980.

Lata, Prem. *Mystic Saints of India: Shankara.* Delhi: Sumit Publications, 1982.

Love, Robert. *The Great Oom: The Improbable Birth of Yoga in America.* New York: Viking, 2010.

Mallinson, James, trans. *Gheranda Samhita.* Woodstock, NY: Yogavidya.com, 2004. http://www.yogavidya.com/Yoga/GherandaSamhita.pdf (accessed April 27, 2016).

Mather, Cotton. "India Christiana." http://quod.lib.umich.edu/e/evans/N01899.0001.001?rgn=main;view=fulltext (accessed April 29, 2016).

Menon, Ramesh. *The Ramayana: A Modern Retelling of the Great Indian Epic.* New York: North Point Press, 2001.

Newcombe, Suzanne. "The Institutionalization of the Yoga Tradition: 'Gurus' B. K. S. Iyengar and Yogini Sunita in Britain." In *Gurus of Modern Yoga*, edited by Mark Singleton and Ellen Goldberg. Oxford: Oxford University Press, 2014. E-book.

Olivelle, Patrick, trans. *Upaniṣads*. New York: Oxford University Press, 1996.

Oman, John Campbell. *The Mystics, Ascetics, and Saints of India: A Study of sadhuism, with an Account of the Yogis, Sanysasis, Bairagis, and Other Strange Hindu Sectarians*. London: T. Fisher Unwin, 1905.

Panikkar, Raimundo, ed. and trans. *The Vedic Experience, Mantramañjarī: an Anthology of the Vedas for Modern Man and Contemporary Celebration*. Berkeley: University of California Press, 1977.

Pennington, Brian K. *Was Hinduism Invented? Britons, Indians, and the Colonial Construction of Religion*. Oxford: Oxford University Press, 2005. E-book.

Pinch, William R. *Warrior Ascetics and Indian Empires*. New York: Cambridge University Press, 2012.

Prabhavananda, Swami, and Christopher Isherwood, trans. *Shankara's Crest-jewel of Discrimination (Viveka-Chunamani)*. 3rd ed. Hollywood, CA: Vedanta Press, 1978. First edition 1947.

Prasad, Rama, trans. "The Yoga Sūtra." In *A Sourcebook in Indian Philosophy*, edited by Sarvepalli Radhakrishnan and Charles A. Moore, 454-85. Princeton, NJ: Princeton University Press, 1989. First published 1957.

Radha, Swami Sivananda. *Hatha Yoga: The Hidden Language*. Spokane, WA: Timeless, 1996.

Radhakrishnan, Sarvepalli and Charles A. Moore, ed. And trans. "The Laws of Manu." *A Sourcebook in Indian Philosophy*. 172-92. Princeton, NJ: Princeton University Press, 1989. First published 1957.

Radin, Dean. *Supernormal: Science, Yoga, and the Evidence for Extraordinary Psychic Abilities*. New York: Deepak Chopra Books, 2015.

Roig-Franzia, Manuel. "Scandal Contorts Future of John Friend, Anusara Yoga." *The Washington Post*, March 28, 2012, https://www.washingtonpost.com/lifestyle/style/scandal-contorts-future-of-john-friend-anusara-yoga/2012/03/28/gIQAeLVThS_story.html (accessed May 6, 2016).

Ruiz, Fernando Pagés. "Krishnamacharya's Legacy: Yoga's Modern Yoga's Inventor." *Yoga Journal*, August 28, 2007, http://www.yogajournal.com/article/philosophy/krishnamacharya-s-legacy/ (accessed May 6, 2016).

Sarkar, Jadunath. *A History of Dasnami Naga Sannyasis*. 1930. dspace.wbpublibnet.gov.in:8080/jspui/handle/10689/9526 (accessed April 29, 2016).

Singleton, Mark. *Yoga Body: The Origins of Modern Posture Practice*. New York: Oxford University Press, 2010.

Singleton, Mark, and Ellen Goldberg, eds. *Gurus of Modern Yoga*. New York: Oxford University Press, 2014. E-book.

Sivananda, Swami. *Yogic Home Exercises: Easy Course of Physical Culture for Modern Men and Women*. Bombay: D.B. Taraporevala Sons, 1944.

Sjoman, N. E. *The Yoga Tradition of the Mysore Palace*. New Delhi: Abhinav Publications, 1999. PDF. First published 1996.

Strauss, Sarah. *Positioning Yoga: Balancing Acts across Cultures*. New York: Berg, 2005.

Svatmarama, Yogi. *Hatha Yoga Pradipika*. Translated by Pancham Sinh, 1914. http://www.sacred-texts.com/hin/hyp/index.htm (accessed April 27, 2016).

Syman, Stephanie. *The Subtle Body: The Story of Yoga in America*. New York: Farrar, Straus & Giroux, 2010.

Thoreau, Henry David. *Walden: Or, Life in the Woods*. New York: T. Y. Crowell & Co., 1899.

Vasu, Rai Bahadur Srisa Chandra, trans. *Gheranda Samhita*. Delhi: Sri Satguru Publications, 1979. PDF. First published 1914-15. http://hinduonline.co/DigitalLibrary/SmallBooks/GherandaSamhitaSanEng.pdf (accessed May 4, 2016).

Vasu, Rai Bahadur Srisa Chandra, and anonymous, trans. *Siva Samhita*. Assembled by Monroe P. Munro, 2000. E-book. http://nitayoga.com/wp-content/uploads/2013/08/Yoga-Shiva-Samhita.pdf (accessed May 4, 2016).

Vivekananda, Swami. *The Complete Works of Swami Vivekananda*. www.ramakrishnavivekananda.info/vivekananda/complete_works.htm (accessed April 29, 2016).

Walton, Christopher L. "Unitarianism and Early American Interest in Hinduism," 1999. http://www.philocrites.com/essays/hinduism.html (accessed April 29, 2016).

White, David Gordon. *Sinister Yogis*. Chicago: University of Chicago Press, 2009. E-book.

Williamson, Lola. *Transcendent in America: Hindu-Inspired Meditation Movements as New Religion*. New York: New York University Press, 2010.

Woodroffe, John. *Introduction to Tantra Śāstra*. 3rd ed. Madras: Ganesh & Co., 1956. First published 1913.

Woodroffe, John. *Tantrarāja Tantra: A Short Analysis*.
    Madras: Ganesh & Co., 1954.

Yogananda, Paramahansa. *Autobiography of a Yogi*. 13th ed.
    Los Angeles, CA: Self-Realization Fellowship, 1998.
    First published 1946.

Yogananda, Paramahansa. Yogoda or Tissue-Will System of
    Physical Perfection, 1925. E-book.

INDEX

A

abhyasa, 95, 100

Advaita Vedanta, 119-20
  Shankara and, 123-24, 127
  vs. Tantra, 133
  view on karma, 128
  view on living liberation, 130

ahimsa, 107
  according to Sivananda, 237-38

anahata, Om as, 51

anatman, 121–22, 124

anjali mudra, 93, 150

Anusara Yoga, 253

aparigraha, 107, 19

Aranyakas, 30, 33-34, 39, 117, 138

Arjuna, 76-77, 80-83, 85-86, 88

asana, 16, 213
  1930s personal account of, 216–18
  in Hatha Yoga, 159, 161, 165
  as limb of Ashtanga, 107, 110
  list of classic, 163-64
  medicalization of, 232
  as meditation posture, 106, 110, 161, 217
  originally considered mudras, 165, 219
  vs. physical culture, 224-25

ascetic, long-haired. *See* keshins

ascetic warriors, 179-80, 182-84, 230

Ashtanga (Patanjali), 94, 105-12, 140
  bhakti in, 110
  influence on Hatha Yoga, 112, 155
  as Raja Yoga, 199

Ashtanga Vinyasa (Jois), 99, 241

atman, 41
  Buddhist view of, 121
  in Neo-Vedanta, 190
  for Patanjali, 104
  in Upanishads, 40–44, 51, 57-58

I

U

Unitarianism, 187-93
  Ram Mohan Roy and, 189-92
Upanishads, 9, 10, 30, 38-40
  vs. *Bhagavad Gita*, 81-82
  Brahman and atman in, 40-44
  caste and, 60
  definition of yoga in, 89
  mahavakyas of, 44
  maya in, 127
  nondualist metaphysics of, 13, 42
  Om in, 51
  origins of Advaita Vedanta in, 136
  origins of Tantra Yoga in, 136
  origins of Vedanta in, 117-119
  prana in, 51-52
  Purusha in, 79
  Ram Mohan Roy and, 189
  reincarnation in, 47-49
  Shankara and, 131-32
  spiritual practices of, 53
  Transcendentalists and, 193

V

vaishya caste, 28
varnas. *See* caste
Vedanta (*see also* Advaita Vedanta; Neo-Vedanta), 43, 115-
    20, 125, 129
Vedas, 10, 19, 23-24
  creation myths in, 25-28
  date of origin of, 22–23
  definition of yoga in, 8
  deities in, 63-64
  lineage of, 33
  as mantras, 148
  maya in, 127
  mystics in, 29-33
  nondualist metaphysics in, 13
  Om in, 51